BOSTON COLLOQUIUM ON
CARDIAC PACING

BOSTON COLLOQUIUM
ON
CARDIAC PACING

edited by

J. WARREN HARTHORNE
(Boston)

HILBERT J. TH. THALEN
(Groningen)

SPRINGER-SCIENCE+BUSINESS MEDIA, B.V. 1977

ISBN 978-94-010-1102-0   ISBN 978-94-010-1100-6 (eBook)
DOI 10.1007/978-94-010-1100-6

© 1977 Springer Science+Business Media Dordrecht
Originally published by Martinus Nijhoff 1977
Softcover reprint of the hardcover 1st edition 1977

FOREWORD

On Friday, the 8th of October 1976, a one day Symposium on Cardiac Pacing, supported by an educational grant from Vitatron Medical, was held at the Sheraton Boston Hotel in Boston, Massachusetts. The intent of the Organizing Committee was to provide a concentrated overview of various aspects of cardiac pacemaker technology ranging from historical aspects, indications, electrode design, energy sources, engineering concepts, detection of malfunction and followup of implanted systems. A look into future trends was also emphasized. The audience consisted of physicians from all parts of the United States with a special interest in pacemaker systems. Their comments, questions, and description of their own experiences, which arose during the discussion period at the end of the program, extended the breadth of the information provided.

J. WARREN HARTHORNE

ACKNOWLEDGEMENT

The editors of this Colloquium on Cardiac Pacing (J.W.H. and H.J.Th.T.) acknowledge the patient understanding and support of their wives, Christa and Ilse through the long hours at night and weekends during which these proceedings were made ready for publication. A special note of appreciation is extended to Dr. Harthorne's secretary, Miss Stephanie Ann Murray, who transcribed the original tape-recorded presentations and typed and retyped the many corrected versions thereafter – all done without complaint and with ultimate good humor.

CONTENTS

CONTRIBUTORS

David L. Bowers, BSEE, Consultant Medical Electronics, 1027 170th Place N.E., Bellevue, WA 98008, USA.

Josef Cywinski, Ph.D., Medical Engineering Department, Massachusetts General Hospital, Boston, MA 02114, USA.

Myrvin H. Ellestad, M.D., Memorial Hospital Medical Center of Long Beach, Long Beach, CA, USA.

Lawrence Gilbert, M.D., Department of Surgery, Newark Beth Israel Medical Center, Pacemaker Center, New Jersey Medical School, Newark, N.J., USA

J. Warren Harthorne, M.D., Massachusetts General Hospital, Boston, MA 02114, USA.

Werner Irnich, Ph.D., RWTH, Abteilung Innere Medizin I, Goethestr. 27-29, 51 Aachen, Federal Republic of Germany.

Marjorie Manhardt, Department of Surgery, Newark Beth Israel Medical Center, Pacemaker Center, New Jersey Medical School, Neward N.J., USA.

John D. Messenger, M.D., Memorial Hospital Medical Center of Long Beach, Long Beach, CA, USA.

George Meyers, Ph.D., Department of Surgery, Newark Beth Israel Medical Center, Pacemaker Center, New Jersey Medical School, Newark, NJ, USA.

Victor Parsonnet, M.D., Department of Surgery, Newark Beth Israel Medical Center, Pacemaker Center, New Jersey Medical School, Newark, N.J., USA.

Thomas Preston, M.D., PHS Hospital, 131 4th Street, Seattle, WA 98114, USA.

Hilbert J. Th. Thalen, M.D., State University Hospital, 59 Oostersingel, Groningen, The Netherlands.

Paul M. Zoll, M.D., Beth Israel Hospital, Boston, MA, USA.

Richard I. Zucker, M.D., Department of Surgery, Newark Beth Israel Medical
    Center, Pacemaker Center, New Jersey Medical School, Newark, N.J., USA.

EARLY HISTORY OF CARDIAC PACING

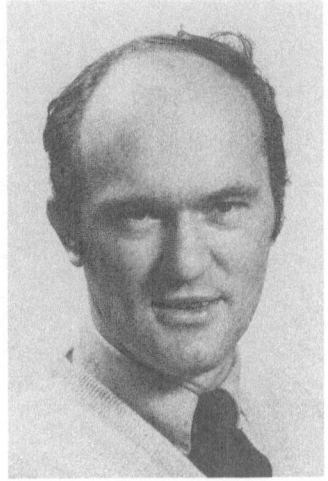

Dr. Hilbert J. Th. Thalen was born April 29, 1939. He studied Medicine at the Medical School of the State University of Groningen where he carried out research for three years in the Laboratory for Medical Physics on pacemaker electrode design, pacemaker circuit design and followup equipment. His doctoral thesis in 1969 entitled 'The Artificial Cardiac Pacemaker: Its History, Development, and Clinical Application' has become a standard international reference textbook and is in its fourth printing. He received his medical degree in 1969. In 1973 he organized the Fourth International Symposium on Cardiac Pacing held at Groningen in The Netherlands. His cardiology training was further extended by a clinical and research appointment at the Massachusetts General Hospital in Boston in 1974-1975. Since 1975, he has been in charge of the Pacemaker Clinic at University Hospital in Groningen, The Netherlands, and carries on an active cardiology practice involving the care of pre- and post-operative cardiac surgical patients. He is a widely traveled lecturer, the author of many papers on various aspects of cardiac pacing, a Fellow of the American College of Cardiology and serves on the editorial boards of the European Journal of Cardiology, Pace, Pacing and Clinical Electrophysiology, and the International Society of Cardiac Pacing. As a longstanding enthusiast of sports medicine, he is cardiac consultant to the Dutch Society of Sports Medicine.

EARLY HISTORY OF CARDIAC PACING

HILBERT J. TH. THALEN, M.D.

An important part of the history of cardiac pacing dates back to Boston. It seems therefore appropriate that a Colloquium in Boston where it all began should include some history. When we speak about history, we not only go back 200 years as with the Bicentennial, but much farther to the first drawing of the heart known to mankind (Fig. 1). It was made 50,000 years before Christ in a Grotto in Altamira in Spain. The drawing not only pictures the heart roughly as we know it today, but it also was positioned well in the body of the animal. This was no coincidence. The people who made the drawing were hunters, and they had to

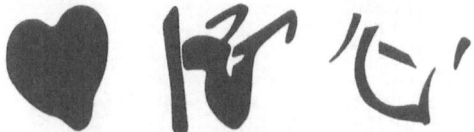

Figure 1. Earliest representation of the heart: (a) Aurignacian (Upper Paleolithic) painting, ca. 50,000 B.C., in red ochre, from the Cave of Pindal in Altamira, Spain; (b) Egyptian hieroglyph, ca 1950, B.C. from the Edwin Smith Papyrus, Line 7, Column 1; (c) Ancient Chinese ideogram (after Dr. I. Veith).

know where to hit the animal most effectively. The heart was known to be important. Greek people called the heart the 'Acropolis of the Body'. Aristotle did research on the functioning of the heart and the heart beat of chicken embryos. Galen, a famous medical researcher and practitioner in Roman times analyzed the function of the heart and the correlation between the various heart compartments. His partly incorrect concept of the function of the heart and the peripheral pulse dominated the medical scene for over fifteen centuries. This persisted until 1628 when Harvey in England wrote his famous De Motu Cordis that brought us the modern concepts of circulation and the heart.

It's not only the anatomy and physiology of the heart, but also the analysis of the peripheral pulse that plays an important role in the history of cardiac pacing. The Greeks, and even before them, the Chinese, often attempted to explain the origin and variations of the pulse. As early as 280 B.C. Wang Chu Ho in China wrote ten books on the pulse. The pulse in Greek is Sphygmos and Sphygmology is the knowledge of the peripheral pulse. It was again Galen, who in Roman times, in his Omni-Opera, interpreted the various pulses. He thought, as did a lot of the people during that time, that every organ had its own pulse and pulse frequency, and every disease had its own pulse pattern. It was again the important work of Harvey in 1628 that outlined our concepts of circulation and peripheral pulse. In the analysis of the pulse at that time there was one problem. It was very difficult to count the pulse. Pulse counting was done in relation to the respiration of the patient or of the doctor himself (Fig. 2). The Greeks and Romans worked with a

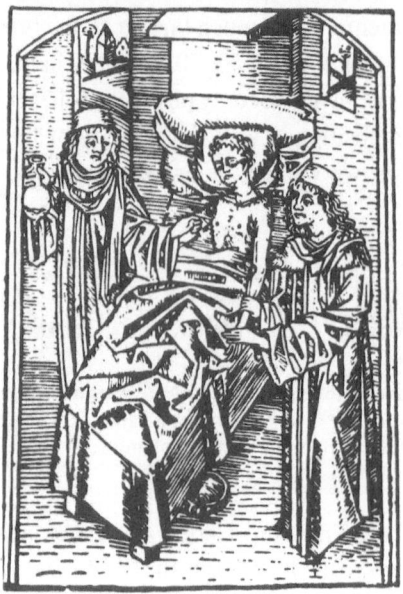

Figure 2. Medieval manuscript on tactile sphygmology from The Netherlands.

water clock, and it was Galileo Galilei who saw a candelabra swinging in the dome of Pisa and found that the frequency of this candelabra was exactly the frequency of his own pulse. He constructed a device called the pulsilogon (Fig. 3) with a heavy ball on a cord. This ball could be fixed at various altitudes along the cord correlating with various frequencies of the swinging cord and ball. By arranging the ball such that the swing correlated with the patient's heart beat, one could read off the frequency of the heart from the altitude of the ball. It was this that initiated the use of the pendulum and ended up in 1657 with Christian Huygens making his first pendulum clock. This pendulum of Christian Huygens was not accurate enough for pulse counting. It was not until 1707, when Floyer in England introduced what he called the 'physicians's pulse watch' that accurate counting of the pulse became possible. By the end of the 18th century, people were able to count the pulse, and they knew especially because of Harvey's contributions how the circulation functioned.

At this same this time people also started to record the pulse with special devices. These systems, called sphygmographs, produced the first recordings of

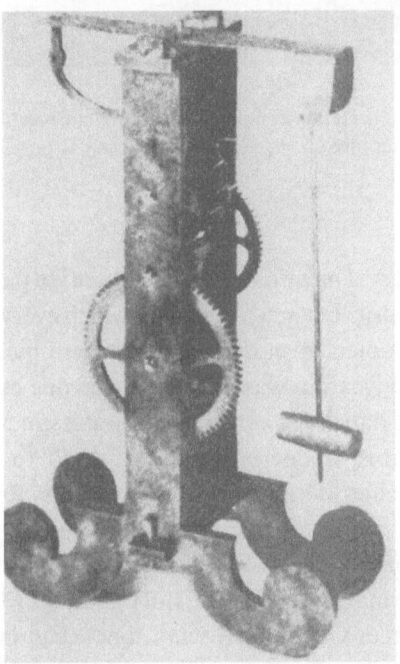

Figure 3. Galilei's Pulsilogon.

the heart beat (Fig. 4). The first recording of a heart beat was made in 1875 by Galaban who did not recognize the phenomenon (Fig. 5).

When one starts counting the pulse, one soon finds out that some heart rates

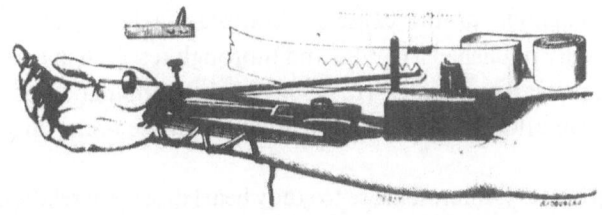

Figure 4. Sphygmographic apparatus based on direct mechanical sensing of pulsations and their transmission by levers.

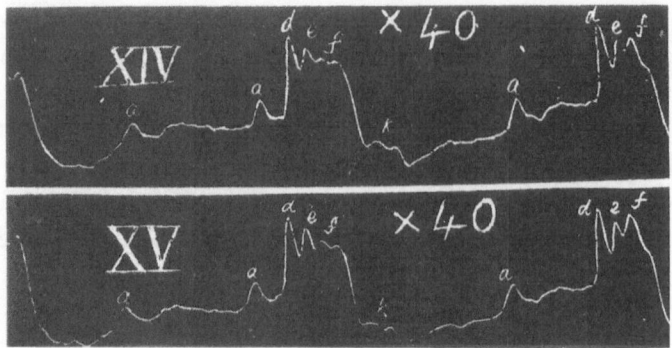

Figure 5. The first graphic documentation of heart block in a tracing recorded in 1875 by Galaban who did not recognize the significance.

go fast and some go slow. As I mentioned already, there is a pulse irregularity and Galen described in his Pulsus Dogma a system in which every organ had its own pulse. The changes promoted in pulse frequency were mostly thought to be caused by emotions; bradycardia was thought to be due especially to mental depression and also to Melancholia. An interesting story in the Greek literature described that Erasistratus, a doctor from Kos, had to look after Prince Antiochus. Prince Antiochus was mentally depressed, and Erasistratus checked his pulse and had all the people of the court walking by. He found out that the pulse of Prince Antiochus increased when his stepmother passed by. He advised that the couple should be married and as the story goes, the Melancholia and the slow heart rate were cured. Galen, in Roman times, had another system. He couldn't have all the people coming around, so he called the names of people involved in personal contacts with his patients and tried to find out if there was some reaction on the pulse. In Burton's Anatomy of Melancholy, this phenomenon is described as "pulsus amatorius". In 1719 Gerbezius in Italy published a very good clinical survey of the pulse. In some of his patients he thought the pulse abnormalities were due to hypochondria. Cheyne in England, known from the Cheyne-Stokes attacks, also had the same thinking. The concept of hypochondria and melancholia as the cause of bradycardia lasted until 1761 when Morgagni in Italy published a careful and thorough research in a case of bradycardia with a priest from Padua. He described the combination of bradycardia and epileptiform attacks and stated that changes in the brain caused the pulse arrhythmias.

By the 19th century, interest arose to study heart disease in relation to diet and body habitus. In this direction in 1827, Robert Adams did a post mortem on a 60 year old officer, and he changed Morgagni's thesis and for the first time mentioned that perhaps the brain was not the cause of the bradycardia, but suggested that the fatty degenerated heart which he found in this general was the cause of the bradycardia and also of the cerebral disease. He was attacked by a lot of people; Mayo from England, Addison, etc. These criticisms were reviewed in 1846 by William Stokes. He had his own experiences and went to the literature and concluded that the concept of Adams was correct that the heart was the cause of the bradycardia. Some years later in a publication in 1890 and in his famous textbook on Cardiology from 1899 Huchard in France described the syndrome of bradycardia and syncopal attacks caused by the diseased heart and proposed to name this disease La Maladie de Adams-Stokes or the Stokes-Adams Disease. In Europe it is called the Stokes Adams Disease after a German publication from the end of the 19th century (Fig. 6).

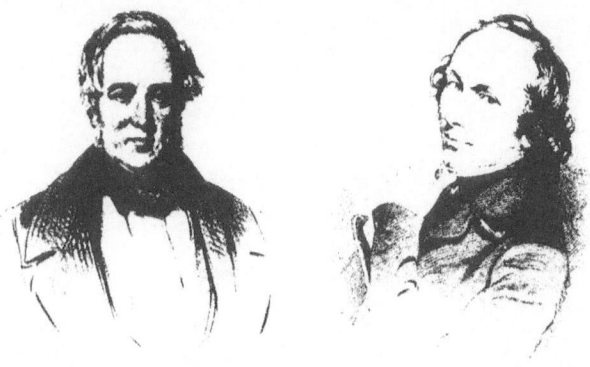

Figure 6. Robert Adams (L) and William Stokes (R): Two of the many physicians who described the disease that bears their name.

Thus, the relation between the circulation, the pulse abnormalities, and the disease had been made. However, the real anatomical substrate was not yet found. In Greek times, Aristotle had watched the heart of chicken embryos. He registered various heart movements and already was able to make a distinction between the atrial and the ventricular contractions. Galen, the Roman, evaluated these findings further and found that the right atrium was the first part of the heart where the contractions started, primum oriens, and also the last part which stopped beating, ultimum moriens. Harvey described in his studies the complete sequence of the contraction as we know now. That was in 1628. In the 19th century Stahnius in 1850 was able to dissect the atrium from the ventricle and Gaskel in 1883 showed us that it was possible to make an interruption between the atria and the ventricles. Physiologists continued this research and John

McWilliams in England wrote in 1807, 'The contraction arises from the heart, the first contraction most probably at the terminal portions of the great veins or close to it.'

The physiologists had spoken. They had made recordings but still there was no anatomic substrate. Of course in 1839, Purkinje in Brno had found his Purkinje fibers, but further discoveries of the conduction system of the heart had to wait until 1893 when His in Germany published his studies on a rabbit heart where he had found with his anatomical studies a tissue connection between the atria and the ventricles, the bundle of His (Fig. 7). The picture of the anatomy cleared further in 1896 when Aschoff and Tawara described the AV node and Tawara

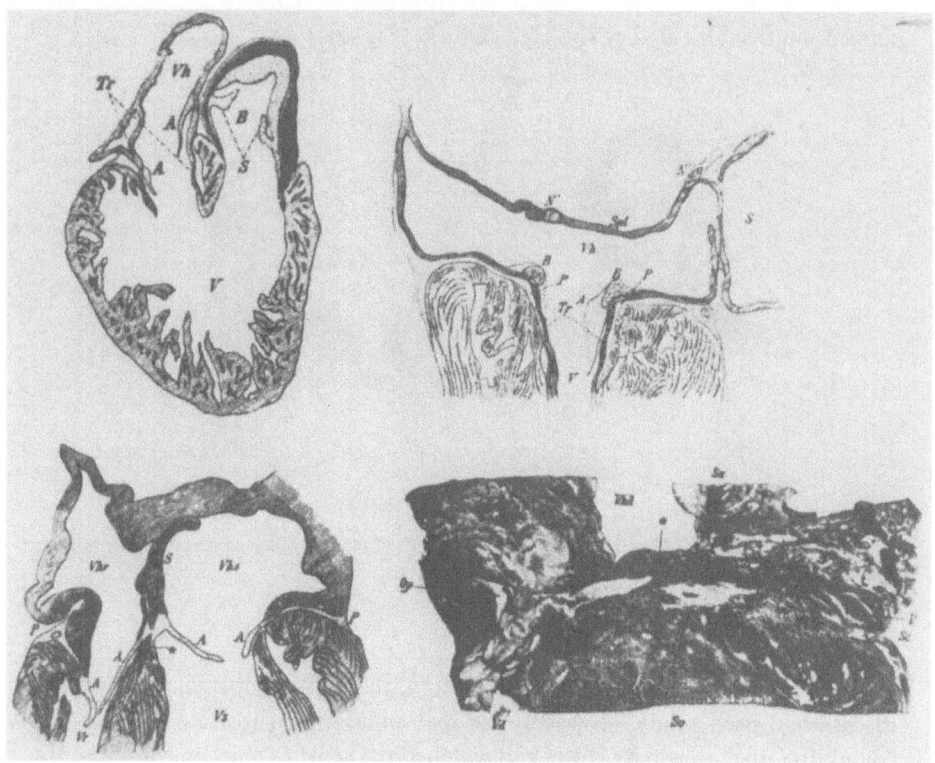

Figure 7. His' original illustrations of the atrio-ventricular node.

traced that the AV node was connected with the Purkinje system via the various bundle branches. In 1907, Keith and Flack in England found what they called the Primum mobile, where everything starts, exactly where the physiologist, McWilliams had thought it to be, the sinus node. The atrial pathways were discussed and described during the first half of our century.

The disease we speak about, atrioventricular block, was already mentioned by His in 1894. He postulated that since the AV bundle connects the atria and ventricles, it could be the cause of the Adams Stokes attacks when interrupted. He did not publish it at that time but only in 1933 and by that time electrocardiography had been developed. The first electrocardiographic tracing of total AV block was made in 1906 by Einthoven in Leiden (Fig. 8) in the Netherlands. From these tracings, Lewis and other people in England became aware that the AV conduction system was the origin of AV block.

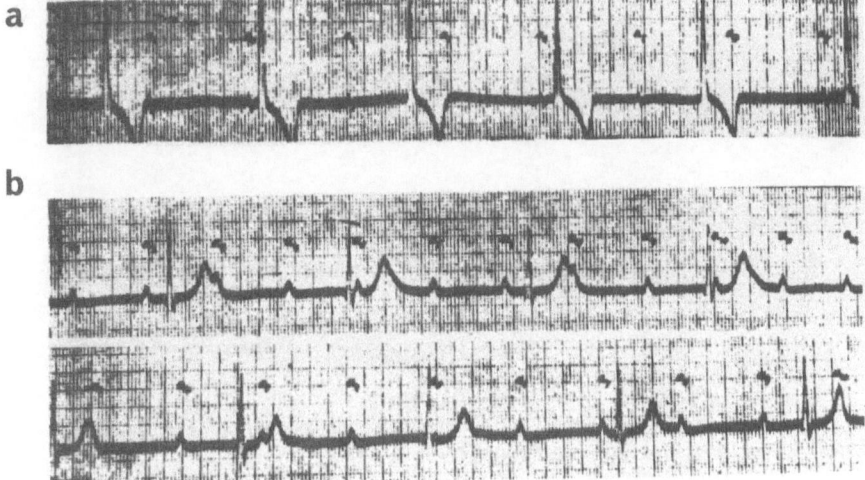

Figure 8. The first electrocardiogram of experimental and clinical heart block shown in Einthoven's classic 1906 paper.

So we have the anatomic substrate, the physiological analysis, and we had the relation between the circulation and the pulse. How did people treat this disease? It was known since the 18th century that you could stimulate the heart. In 1804 Aldini described studies in Tur (Italy) where they stimulated the heart of decapitated criminals with the column of Galvani and Volta. Electricity started in the 18th century and was applied especially for indirect stimulation of various organs, among others, to speed up the heart frequency. Galvanization became popular, and various devices were developed in the 18th and 19th centuries. It was known that through stimulation of the sympathetic nerves (Fig. 9), the heart rhythm could be influenced as a sphygomograph tracing recording of that time by Beard demonstrated (Fig. 10). There were even special clinics in the 18th and 19th century for electrical treatment and cardiac stimulation, like the clinic of Charcot seen in Figure 11. These clinics were rather popular and originated the development of various devices like sophisticated units for a doctor's office and also special patient devices to use at their own home.

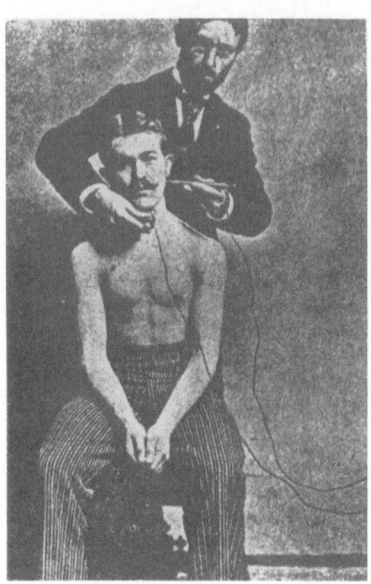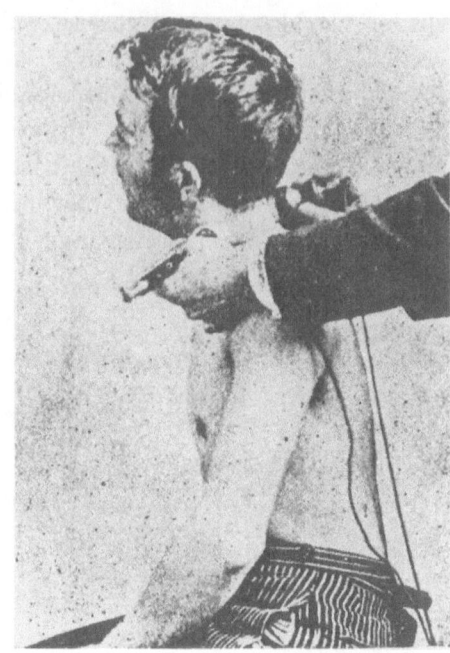

Figure 9. Techniques for stimulating vagal and cervical sympathetic nerves. These modalities were extensively practiced for a wide assortment of chest diseases.

Galvanic stimulation became popular in the 18th and 19th century. Many theories concerning the exact stimulation procedure were published. Increasing the heart rate of a slow beating heart by indirect stimulation was known but the technique of direct stimulation of the heart and also stimulation of an arrested heart as with the investigations of Aldini was difficult. Perhaps acupuncture, already popular in the 19th century started another direct approach to the heart; a needle electrode driven into the heart through the intact chest. Later the needle

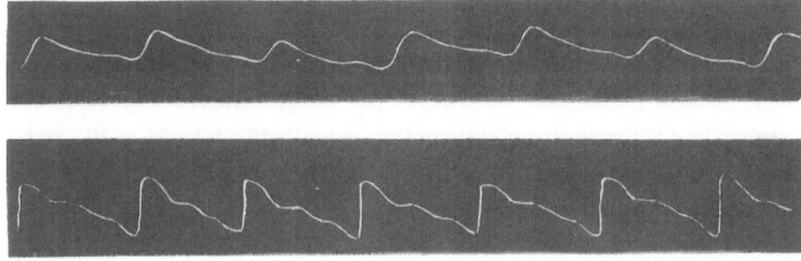

Figure 10. Sphygmographic records made by Beard showing a normal pulse (upper) and alterations provoked by galvanization or faradization of cervical sympathetic nerves in normal subjects (lower).

was replaced by a hollow needle through which drugs could be introduced into the heart. Hyman in New York, analyzed the various ways of stimulation of the heart in 1932 and concluded that most probably it's not the drug that stimulates a stopped heart, but the needle puncture per se. He developed a device (Fig. 12) with a needle electrode that could be put through the chest into the heart which produced interrupted pulses and not Galvanic current as used earlier. The device had a spring mechanism which had to be rewound every six minutes. This enabled Hyman to save the lives of at least two patients for 24-48 hours in 1932. Hyman, the man who really started cardiac pacing, also gave it its name, as he wrote: 'Since this apparatus is a substitute for the non-functioning normal sinus nodal pacemaker, it is called the artificial pacemaker.' It took, however, about twenty years before cardiac pacing achieved its present day acceptance.

The modern era of cardiac pacing started in Boston. It was in Boston in 1950 that Callaghan and Bigelow of Toronto presented a report on stimulation of the sinus node in a dog. Their stimulation unit looked a little bit like the external stimulator we have now. There was a Bostonian in the audience who remembered this presentation and used it clinically. By November, 1952 he published in the New England Journal of Medicine his experience with stimulation of the heart of two patients with an external stimulator and skin electrodes. Other groups followed like Schwedel and Furman, who applied a transvenous catheter with an external unit that could be pushed by the patient on a small cart. The patient had a wire of twenty meters to enable some activities.

Further development of electrodes and electronics – especially the development of transistors enabled Elmqvist, the engineer, and Senning, the surgeon, to construct the first implantable unit clinically applied in October 1958 in a patient who at this time is still alive (Fig. 14). The unit of Elmqvist and Senning used rechargeable batteries. In the USA, Greatbatch and Chardack and other groups in Europe developed pacemakers with ordinary batteries. A lot of energy was stored in these relatively large units.

Now, fifteen years later, we are talking about newer units with the longer lasting cells that enable implantation periods of about ten years. These developments will be discussed at this colloquium, but we thought it useful to give you an outline of how everything started. It's a short outline but we think that before we go into the details of the newer developments that Paul Zoll, the man who started everything in Boston and around the world, and who is present here should tell you himself what he did in 1950 and how things developed later.

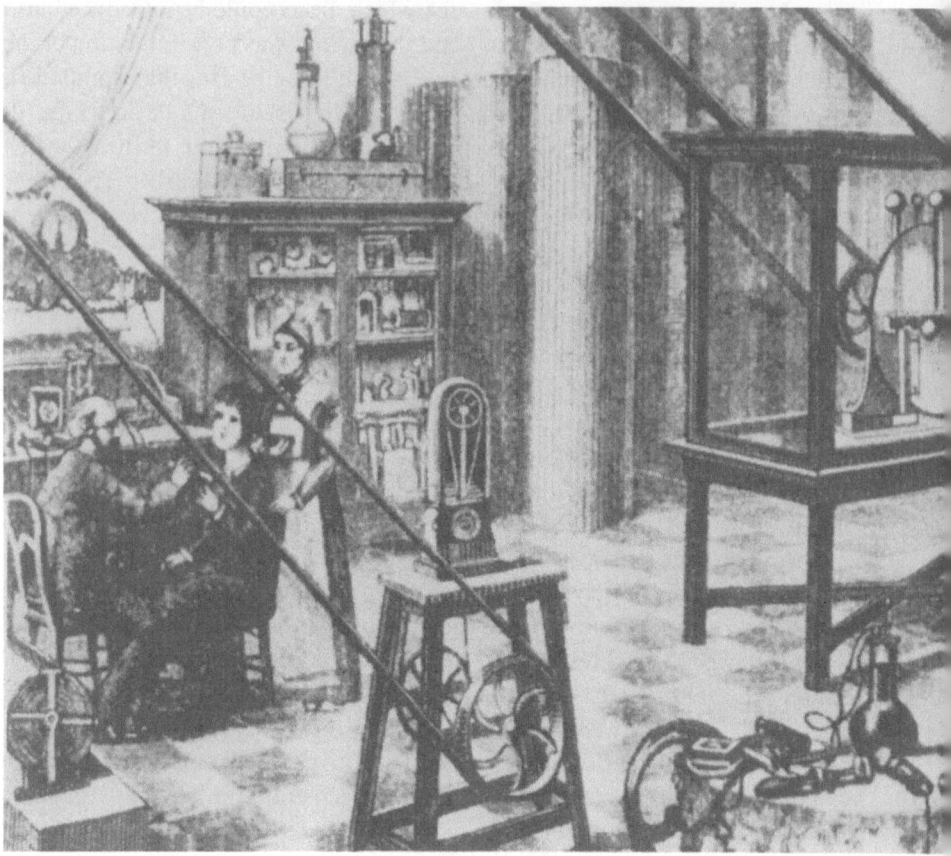

Figure 11. The electrotherapy clinic of Charcot. At left, a fully dressed patient is being stimulated across the precordium.

Figure 12. Albert Hymans' artificial cardiac pacemaker (1932).

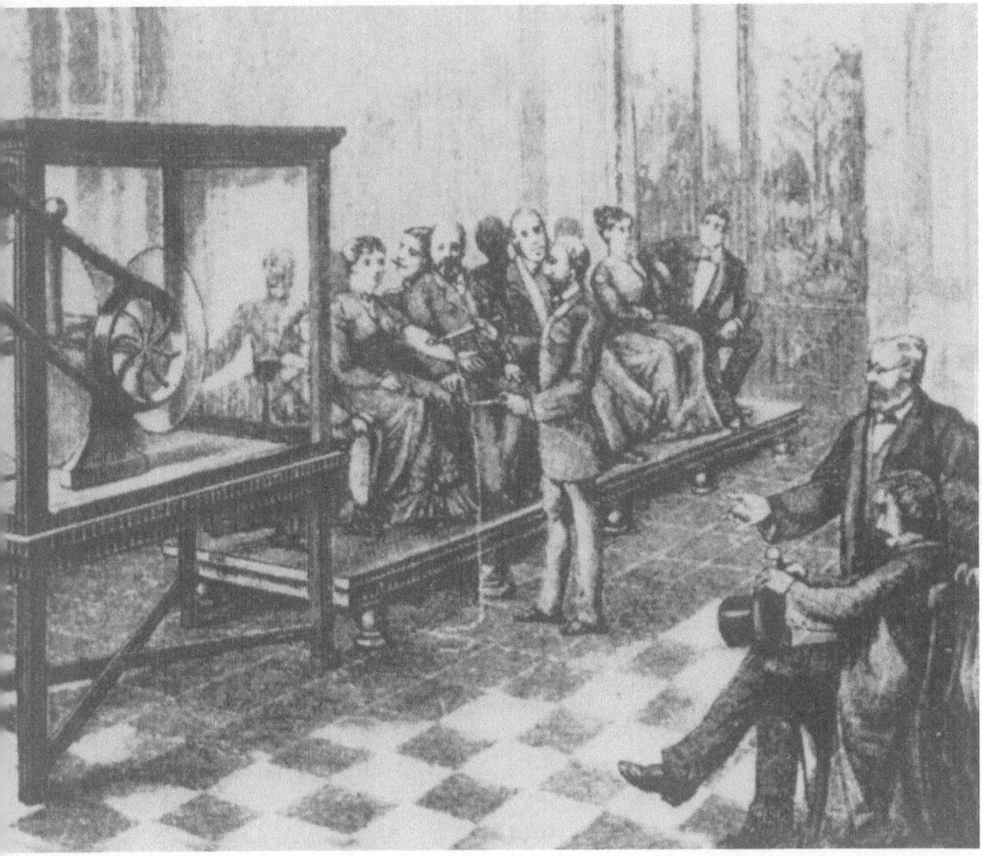

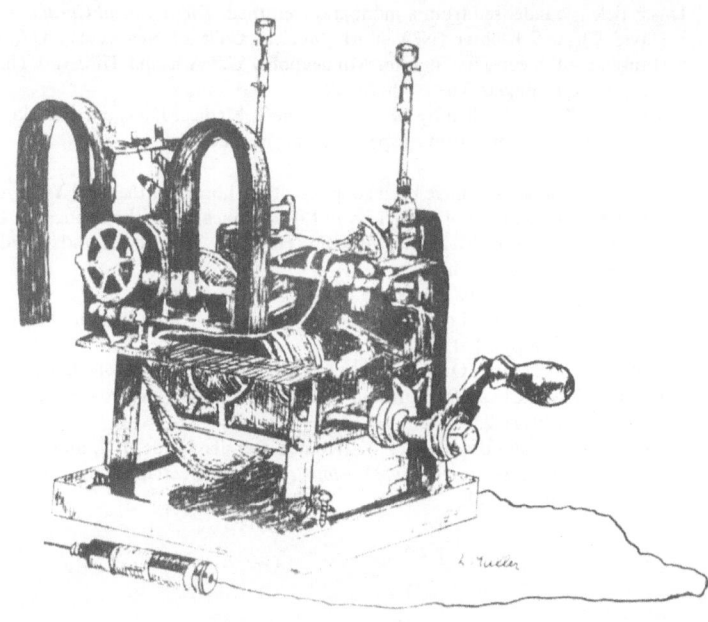

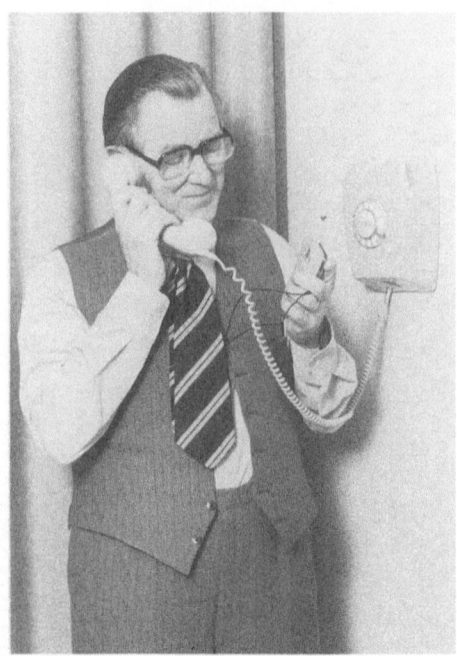

Figure 14. Mr. Arne H.W. Larsson, the first patient to receive an implantable pacemaker in October, 1958 by Dr. Elmqvist and Dr. Senning in Stockholm (Sweden) checking his 23rd pacemaker during a recent visit at the Pacemaker Clinic of the University of Groningen (The Netherlands).

Literature

This article is condensed from a monograph entitled: *The Artificial Cardiac Pacemaker History* by David Chas. Schechter (New York Medical College, New York, U.S.A.), Dennis Stillings (Museum of Electricity in Life, Minneapolis, U.S.A.), and Hilbert J.Th. Thalen (University Hospital, Groningen, The Netherlands).
The book will be published by Martinus Nijhoff, Medical Division, The Hague, The Netherlands as part of a series on various aspects of Cardiac Pacing.

Data for the publication have been collected at the library of the New York Academy of Medicine (New York), Museum of Electricity in Life (Minneapolis), the Francis A. Countway Library of Medicine (Boston), the Teyler Museum (Haarlem, The Netherlands), and the Museum of the University of Groningen.
Selected references on this subject by the above authors are:
Schechter, David Chas., Lillehei, C. Walter and Soffer, Alfred, History of Heart Block. *Diseases of the Chest* 55, Suppl. 1, 1969.
Schechter, David Chas., Origins of Electrotherapy. *New York State J. Med.* 71, 11-12, 1971.
Schechter, David Chas., Background of Clinical Cardiac Electrostimulation. *New York State J. Med.* 71-72, 1971/72.
Thalen, H.J.Th., and den Berg, J.W., Homan van der Heide, J.N. and Nieveen, J., *The Artificial Cardiac Pacemaker, its History, Development and Clinical Application.* Royal Van Gorcum, Assen 1969, 3rd printing 1975.

THE INTERMEDIATE HISTORY
OF CARDIAC PACING

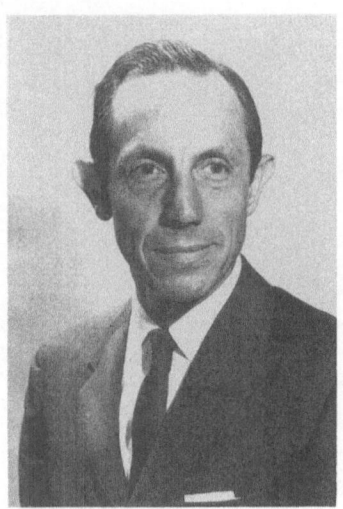

Dr. Paul M. Zoll holds the rank of Clinical Professor of Medicine at Harvard Medical School and Physician at the Beth Israel Hospital, Boston, Massachusetts. His many contributions as an active investigator and early pioneer in the development of electrical stimulation of the heart have gained him the identity as the 'father' of modern cardiac pacing.

THE INTERMEDIATE HISTORY
OF CARDIAC PACING

PAUL M. ZOLL, M.D.

I must admit to some embarrassment about writing about the intermediate history of cardiac pacemakers because my view is necessarily a personal one. I will tell about myself a good deal, so I wish to apologize for giving this rather slanted view.

Back in 1948 after World War II, cardiac stimulation for high degree AV block or cardiac arrest was a rather difficult problem. Stokes Adams disease, as you heard, was known then. It wasn't a very common disease and was not well understood. It was supposed to occur infrequently in the elderly and it had a very bad prognosis; 50 percent of patients were dead within a year after their first Stokes Adams attack, and in many the first attack was fatal. Treatment was also not very satisfactory. Drug treatment was widely used. We gave atropine, ephedrine or epinephrine in those days. The major drug therapy was studied by Ray Gilchrist in Edinburgh in the 1930's. His demonstrations that these drugs increased the idioventricular rate by several beats per minute was the basis of our therapeutic attempts. Epinephrine was given by intracardiac or intravenous injection in doses which we thought in those days were reasonable, 0.10-.30 cc of a 1:1000 solution. In other words, from 100-300 micrograms were given in one bolus, amounts that we now recognize as really very large. These doses certainly contributed to the mortality of patients undergoing emergency treatment.

Similarly, cardiac arrest in those days was a difficult matter. Treatment followed the tenets presented by Claude Beck in 1947 of emergency thoracotomy under any circumstances, direct cardiac massage or compression to squeeze blood out of the heart to the brain, and countershock defibrillation directly on the exposed heart. His work was based on the preceding very careful studies by Carl Wiggers in Cleveland. Some of you may be old enough to remember that our cardiologists carried large jack knives and even our poor eye surgeons were taken to the dog laboratories and shown how to cut chests open under emergency situations. It was a difficult time for all.

As you have heard, Dr. Albert S. Hyman had presented a technique of percutaneous electric stimulation of the heart in 1930 and 1932. I might add another personal note here. I knew Dr. Hyman; he used to sit in the front row at the heart meetings. With his impressive manner, gray moustache, and Van Dyke beard he would stand up and object to many of the so-called new advances that were presented. Furthermore, his brother, who has been a patient of mine here in Boston, just spent two months in the hospital with an abrupt episode of cardiac arrest, ventricular fibrillation, and prolonged absence of ventricular rhythmicity. He suffered through all the complications of emergency cardiac resuscitation, but has recovered and is home doing well.

In 1948 Herman Hellerstein and Liebow in Cleveland presented a technique of thermal stimulation or acceleration of the heart by passing a 'thermode,' a glass U-tube attached to a pervenous catheter into the right atrium by which they warmed the endocardial surface of the right atrium and accelerated atrial rhythmicity. This is a technique of thermal acceleration, you might say. We also have recently worked on this idea. Cardiac warming offers considerable value in special applications in improving and accelerating cardiac rhythmicity. This was the background in 1950 when I became interested in external electric stimulation because, as Claude Beck used to say, 'These hearts were too good to die.' They were perfectly capable of effective contractions; they just didn't get the stimulus to do so.

We worked in the laboratory following the lead of Bigelow and Callaghan whose presentation I listened to here in 1950 at the American College of Surgeons Meeting. With an external electric pacemaker we stimulated the hearts of dogs in normal sinus rhythm with one electrode in the esophagus and the other one over the precordium. We demonstrated in the laboratory to our own satisfaction that external artificial electric stimulation can provoke effective ventricular beats in dogs with normal sinus rhythm. When we saw the first ventricular extrasystoles on a rotating fluorescent screen attached to an old Sanborn photographic machine, I called in everybody in the laboratory to look also. I think I recognized at that time that a new field of electric cardiac stimulation had begun. I think I foresaw almost all of the implications of what has followed in the next 25 years. Some of the complications and problems I am afraid I didn't recognize then, but I did see the implications for therapeutic progress.

In 1952 indeed, we applied this technique of external electric stimulation to resuscitate two patients from ventricular standstill. The first patient lived only 20 minutes; the second one survived after 52 hours of stimulation. Electric stimulation in the second patient was prolonged because intrinsic ventricular beats were absent at every test interruption of stimulation. We then became rather desperate and uneasy because we did not know what to expect. We were facing the new problem of persistent ventricular standstill, one that had never been met before. Finally, intrinsic ventricular rhythmicity did return after the intramuscular injection of ephedrine.

Another difficulty faced us from many sides. Many people, including my own cardiac fellow, thought that it might be blasphemous, improper, or unethical to keep a patient alive by such artificial means. I must say that I didn't understand that objection then, and I don't understand it now. I was saved from a great deal of embarrassment at the time by a small article in the Catholic weekly newspaper, *The Pilot*. A very favorably minded editor told his parishioners not to worry about this outlandish treatment going on at the Beth Israel Hospital, that God worked in many strange ways and this was one way of His expressing the Divine Will, and therefore it was not blasphemous at all. I took great comfort in being promoted in this way, although I was a little uneasy about my credentials.

Another problem was widespread disbelief in our work. People didn't believe that we were able to stimulate the heart and to provide effective beats. Indeed, the next spring I submitted a project to the United States Public Health Service for the large sum of $ 5,000 to keep our work going for a year or two. It was turned down by the head of the Study Committee, an eminent physiologist from Cleveland, who had done much research in this field many years earlier. He decided our success was not possible because he had tried to do something of this nature some twenty years before and had failed. This disbelief continued for many years thereafter and is still present. The house officers at the hospital tell me time and again that external electric stimulation doesn't work. They know it doesn't work because they were told so in Medical School. People at the scene in episodes of cardiac arrest do not think about external electric stimulation, even though I believe it is a most successful, easily applied, effective means of providing ventricular beats in the emergency of cardiac arrest. This disbelief was bolstered in 1960 by the people at Johns Hopkins who developed the very effective technique of external cardiac massage or compression as an emergency measure in cardiac arrest. They said that external electric stimulation might be useful in Stokes-Adams disease, but it was ineffective otherwise. If, by Stokes Adams disease, they meant ventricular standstill, I would agree with them. They implied that electric stimulation was ineffective unless the patient had high-degree AV block. I believe this to be in error. We demonstrated in 1950 that we could drive the heart in dogs in normal sinus rhythm indefinitely externally with electric stimulation and indeed today we use pacemakers in many kinds of situations that do not involve high degree AV block. This disbelief in electric stimulation has now worn off with respect to direct electric stimulation perhaps, but it still persists for external stimulation.

In 1953 I first presented some of our earlier results at the New England Cardiovascular Society Meeting. One of my close friends, an eminent cardiologist in Boston, told my wife sitting next to him that the external pacemaker was a marvelous little toy and very useful for abstruse studies in the laboratory, but it would be of no clinical value. Stokes-Adams disease, he said, was such an infrequent condition occurring only in the elderly that at best it might briefly prolong the unhappy life of a few patients. It is true that Stokes-Adams disease is unpredictable, potentially lethal, and tends to occur in elderly people, but the wide application of cardiac pacing today I think indicates that it has indeed a very wide clinical usefulness.

The very unpredictability of Stokes-Adams disease and its lethality led us, about 1954, to think about means of turning on our external pacemaker in a more effective and reliable way than having a human being stand by ready to switch on the external pacemaker. Many sad experiences provided the impetus for us to develop a more reliable electronic monitor of cardiac rhythmicity with audible and visual signals of the heart beats, and an automatic alarm signal in the absence of intrinsic beats. A year or so later we extended the idea of external stimulation through the chest wall to the technique of external cardiac counter-shock termination of ventricular fibrillation and other ventricular tachycardias.

At about this time I was working with Dr. Arthur Linenthal, who had, I must admit, a more fundamental view of cardiac rhythmicity and arrhythmias than I had. We demonstrated that one could indeed suppress recurring tachycardias by driving the heart fast enough to wipe them out. This study may be the basis of our present ideas about overdrive suppression of arrhythmias. We also then developed the technique of intravenous administration of dilute solutions of catecholamines, epinephrine and isoproterenol, to arouse, to accelerate, and to maintain ventricular rhythmicity.

In 1957, I was visited by Hughes Day, who pointed out to me what I knew very well, that all the techniques necessary to resuscitate patients from cardiac arrest were available; we had monitors, stimulators, and defibrillators. He asked why these techniques were not being applied to patients with acute myocardial infarction, so many of whom died abruptly in cardiac arrest. I had, indeed, suggested such a program for trial in my hospital. There was, however, some disbelief that such a program would be successful, also a reluctance to undertake the attendant problems. Hughes Day then went on to develop the first Coronary Care Unit and demonstrated a reduction of the incidence of sudden death by half in patients with acute myocardial infarction.

The problems with recurring cardiac arrest in patients with Stokes-Adams disease were known since the second patient whom we treated in 1952. This man was resuscitated, as I told you, initially after 52 hours of continuous stimulation; he then recovered, had no more Stokes-Adams attacks, went home, and after eleven months died abruptly of another Stokes-Adams attack, a demonstration that patients who have had one Stokes-Adams attack must be stimulated continuously for the rest of their lives. To solve this problem we attempted to develop internal long-term electric pacemakers beginning in 1954, and we failed. We were unable to solve the problem of a persistent rise in thresholds for stimulation. The initial thresholds were low, about 1-2 milliamperes with an electrode implanted directly in the myocardium. Over a period of 2 to 8 weeks, however, the thresholds would rise to 20 milliamperes or more so that stimulation would be intolerable. We worked on this problem unsuccessfully I must say with some embarrassment for four or five years. We couldn't figure out why the thresholds rose so high and so irregularly. It wasn't until a small article appeared in the Dow Corning publication about the use of Silastic (silicon rubber) in the human body that we realized the problem was one of a foreign body reaction, not to infection, but to microscopic contamination. We followed the advice that Silas Braley gave in that little article of boiling our electrodes in Ivory flakes and not touching them thereafter, whereupon the problem of rise in threshold disappeared. For about ten years we continued an almost religious ritual of avoiding contamination of our electrodes by this procedure. In present day practice, the same sort of end result is obtained by having the manufacturers of the electrodes clean and sterilize them properly. I think there are still some opportunities for contamination, however, that may account for some of our current instances of so-called exit block.

In 1959 I attended a conference called by RCA at the Rockefeller Institute that was chaired by General Sarnoff in which there was a discussion of long-term cardiac pacing. At that time a long-term electrode was not even available. The best that had been done was by Lillehei, and others in Minneapolis, who had placed electrodes in the myocardium that all failed within 56 days because of rising threshold. That conference was dominated by electronic engineers who were interested in applications of electronics in medicine, and there was a great deal of excited conversation about positive and negative feedback. I don't know what the terms in vogue are at the present time, but in those days feedback was a magic word indeed. Positive feedback meant that the atrial signal would trigger a ventricular stimulus so as to restore AV conduction; negative feedback meant that a ventricular signal would suppress the appearance of a ventricular stimulus. So we had even then the basis for programmable, synchronous, demand, stand-by, etc. pacemakers. I objected, in vain, that we had no way of applying these attractive ideas because at that time we didn't have an effective electrode.

After the meeting Dr. John Schwedel told me that a young surgical house office working in the catheterization laboratory at the Montefiore Hospital, a fellow named Seymour Furman, had developed a technique for long-term stimulation of the heart by passing an endocardial catheter electrode into the right ventricle. I went with him to the hospital late that afternoon and observed the patient whom we saw on a previous slide, who was indeed being stimulated repeatedly for days in this way. I recognized this experience as the beginning of clinical long-term electric stimulation of the heart.

It was a year earlier, in 1958, that Senning in Stockholm had implanted the first long-term electrode, developed by Elmquist, in the myocardium of a patient. In this country Samuel Hunter, a surgical resident of Lillehei in St. Paul, applied the

Hunter-Roth thumbtack electrode in the ventricle for long-term electric stimulation in 1959. We didn't get to put in our first long-term cardiac pacemaker until the following year, July 1960, when we had a patient who demanded it of us even though we still were not ready. The man, a physician in fact, originally from Poland, by way of England and Canada, had suffered repeated Stokes-Adams attacks for a few years. He told us he couldn't wait for us to perfect our instruments. He wanted a pacemaker to be put in at once. We did so. He lived for three years and died of complications of cardiac pacemaking that were so many in those times. Most of these complications have now been solved. They deal with displacement, fracture, and infection of electrodes, with unreliable electronic components and circuitry, with inadequate energy sources, with leaky encapsulation, with every aspect of cardiac pacing. The major progress since those days has been the gradual, painfully slow, increasing reliability of the cardiac pacemaker-electrode system. We still have far to go in this primary task of making pacemakers entirely safe.

Literature

Zoll, P.M., Historical Development of Cardiac Pacemakers. *Progress Cardiovascular Diseases* 14, 421, 1972.
Zoll, P.M., Development of Electric Control of Cardiac Rhythm. *JAMA* 226, 881, 1973.

INDICATIONS FOR VARIOUS TYPES
OF CARDIAC PACEMAKERS

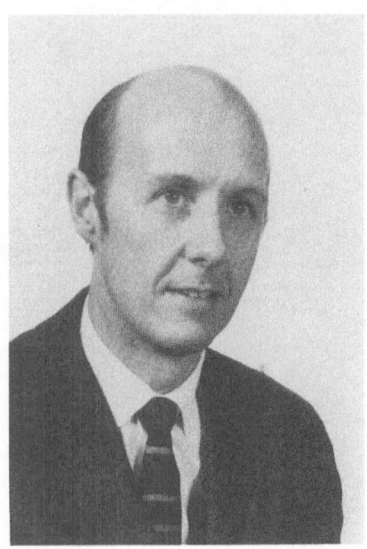

Dr. J. Warren Harthorne received his undergraduate training at Bowdoin College and Medical degree from McGill University School of Medicine. Following internship and two years of residency in Internal Medicine at the Montreal General Hospital, he joined the Cardiac Unit of the Massachusetts General Hospital, Boston, Massachusetts. After three years of Cardiac Fellowship training, he was appointed to the staff in 1965. A long interest in cardiac catheterization led to directing the activities of the Cardiac Catheter Laboratory from 1972 to 1974 with more recent emphasis on transvenous pacemaker procedures. He is on the teaching staff of the Massachusetts General Hospital and Mt. Auburn Hospital and is Assistant Professor of Medicine at Harvard Medical School. He is the author of many papers and abstracts on various topics in cardiology.

INDICATIONS FOR VARIOUS TYPES
OF CARDIAC PACEMAKERS

J. WARREN HARTHORNE, M.D.

As physicians, we have all become accustomed to selecting whatever therapeutic modality best suits the clinical needs presented by our patients. The host of new drugs and mechanical as well as bio-electronic aids introduced in the past ten years has made this a sometimes awesome task. During the seventeen or so years since their introduction, cardiac pacemaker systems have evolved from rather simple fixed rate ventricular stimulators of erratic reliability to sophisticated instruments borne of space age technology and deriving their power from new sources of electrical energy. The busy physician in his day-to-day practice is dazzled by the eloquent and often unsubstantiated claims of competing sales personnel and is at risk of sallying forth in a vain search for an electronic holy grail. Thus, as physicians choosing an electronic pacemaker system which best suits the individual patient's clinical circumstances, there are certain basic principles which are appropriate to emphasize:

Firstly, as in most aspects of medical therapy, it is best not to overtreat the patient, and one must try to match the pacemaker device to the purpose of pacing (Fig. 1).

PURPOSE OF PACING	PREFERRED METHOD
1. PREVENTION OF BRADYCARDIA	VENTRICULAR PACING (DEMAND)
2. PREVENTION OF BRADYCARDIA PLUS AUGMENTATION OF CARDIAC OUTPUT	ATRIAL, A-V SYNCHRONOUS OR A-V SEQUENTIAL PACING
3. OVERDRIVE SUPPRESSION OF ARRHYTHMIAS	ATRIAL PACING
4. INTERRUPTION OF ECTOPIC ARRHYTHMIAS	RAPID ATRIAL PACING, A-V SEQUENTIAL OR VENTRICULAR DEMAND

Figure 1.

The management of simple bradycardia may thus best be handled by ventricular stimulation. The argument over whether fixed rate devices or demand systems should be employed continues to arise despite ten years' experience with each method, and one must balance the greater complexity and slightly shortened generator life of demand systems against the proposed but unsubstantiated claims of the hazards of competitive pacing by fixed rate units in patients with chronic heart block. Figure 2 illustrates the methods available for the management of bradycardia due to heart block. Asynchronous ventricular stimulation is seldom employed due to competition with endogenous rhythms. Ventricular

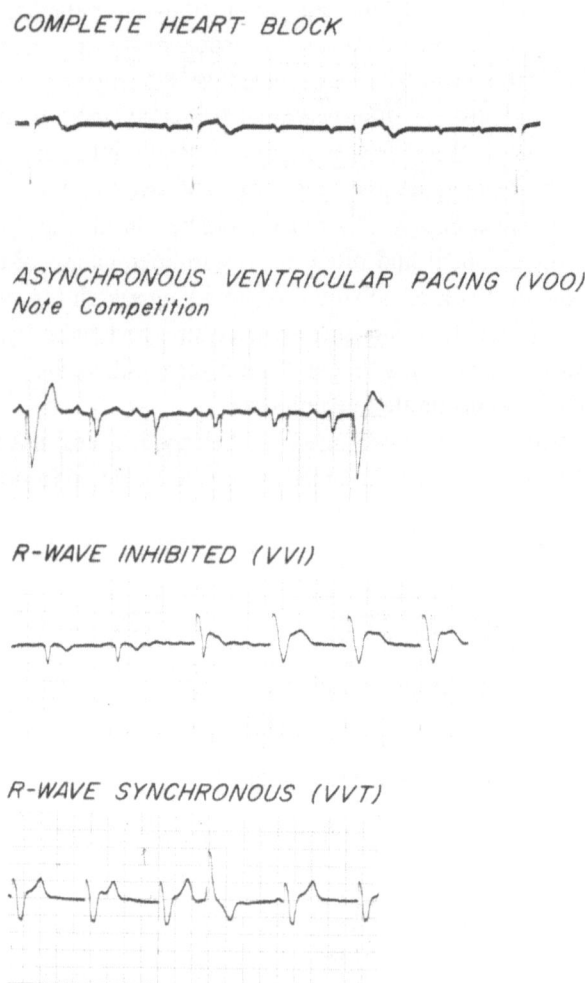

Figure 2. Techniques of ventricular stimulation employed in treatment of bradyarrhythmias. Symbols in brackets refer to international code of pacemaker type.

inhibited demand pacing is the type most commonly employed both for temporary or permanent pacing systems. R-wave synchronous ventricular stimulation also averts competition with intrinsic rhythm by discharge of the pacemaker stimulus into the refractory period of naturally occurring beats in contrast to ventricular inhibited systems in which the output stimulus is suppressed by spontaneous rhythms.

When control of a bradyarrhythmia plus augmentation of the cardiac output is desired, some technique whereby normal atrio-ventricular synchrony can be established is preferred, and, depending upon the underlying conduction tissue abnormality, may be accomplished by atrial pacing, A-V synchronous pacing or A-V sequential pacing. An illustration of these techniques is seen in the accompanying illustrations. The relative merits of ventricular demand pacing vs. atrial stimulation are shown in Fig. 3. There is little question that the reliability and

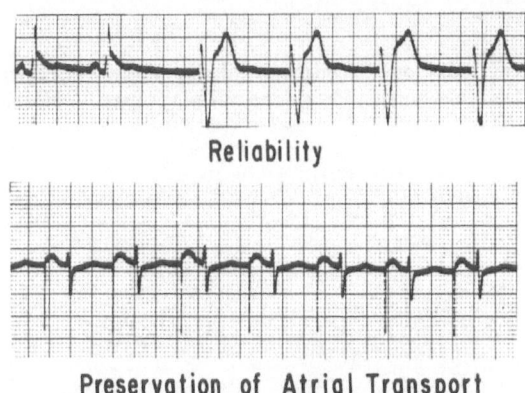

Reliability

Preservation of Atrial Transport

Figure 3.A. Relative merits of ventricular (demand or standby) stimulation versus atrial stimulation.

dependability of ventricular pacemaker electrodes is greater with today's technology. However in individual situations, the physiologic advantages of a properly timed atrial transport mechanism may outweigh the differences in lead system stability. A clinical case in point is demonstrated in Figs. 4 and 5. The patient was an 85 year old lady with Stokes Adams attacks due to sinus node dysfunction. Following establishment of ventricular demand pacing, Stokes Adams attacks continued to recur despite demonstration of dependable R-wave synchronous pacemaker function. Simultaneous recording of intra arterial pressure during the inception of ventricular stimulation revealed a drop of 120 mm Hg with the patient lying down (Fig. 4). Conversion to an atrial pacemaker (Fig. 5) minimized the fall in arterial pressure and interrupted the attacks. A more pressing case for the importance of the atrial transport mechanism is seen in the setting of the acutely ill patient following acute myocardial infarction or car-

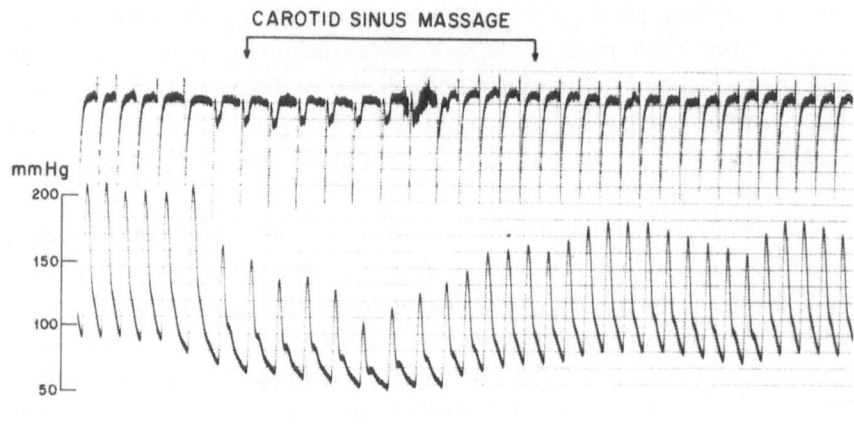

Figure 4. Intra arterial recording of blood pressure during induced ventricular synchronous pacing. The patient, age 82, had sick sinus syndrome and was lying supine during this recording.

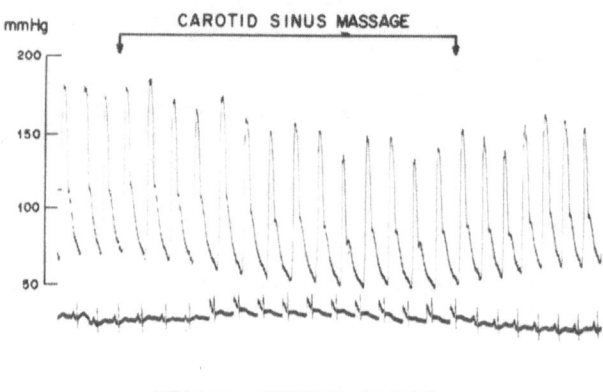

Figure 5. Intra arterial recording of blood pressure of the same patient depicted in Figure 4 following conversion to atrial pacing. Maximum blood pressure drop is 40 mm Hg due to combined effect on heart rate and peripheral resistance of carotid massage.

diopulmonary bypass (Fig. 6). Here the contribution of 20 to 30 mm of higher systolic pressure during atrial stimulation may be of critical importance in sustaining selected organ perfusion as in the kidney.

In patients with disordered atrio ventricular conduction mechanisms wherein varying degrees of A-V block occur with atrial stimulation, more complicated double lead systems are employed with one lead in the atrium and one in the ventricle. When dependable atrial activity is present, the atrial electrode can be used much like an antenna to detect the spontaneously occurring atrial activity

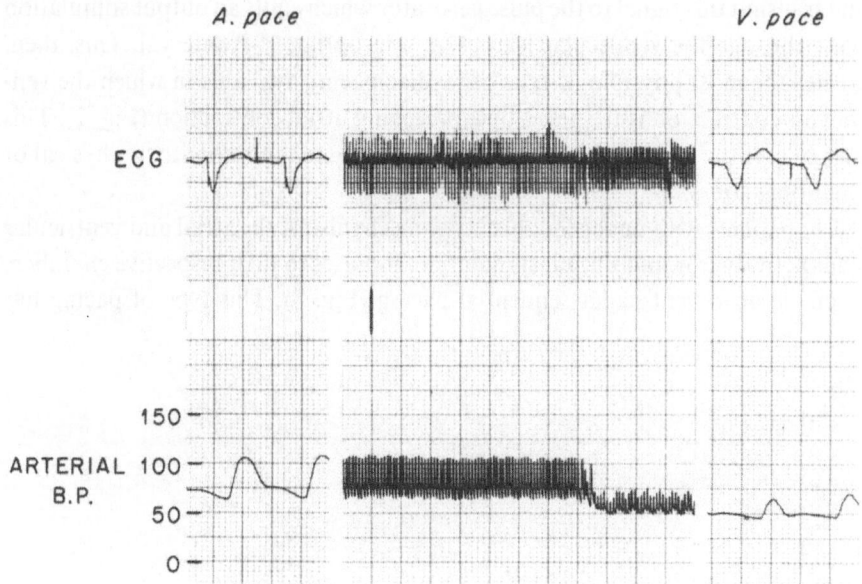

Figure 6. Intra arterial recording of blood pressure in a patient with an extensive myocardial infarction during atrial pacing (left side) and ventricular pacing (right side).

COMPLETE HEART BLOCK
Rate 31/min

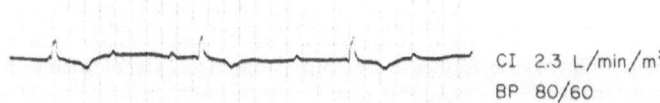

CI 2.3 L/min/m²
BP 80/60

VENTRICULAR PACING
Rate 70/min

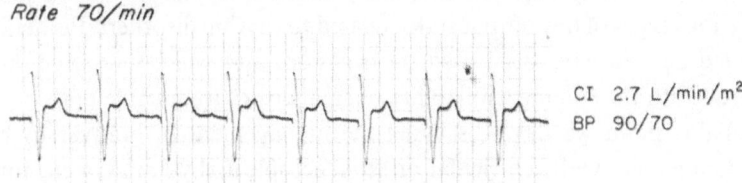

CI 2.7 L/min/m²
BP 90/70

ATRIOVENTRICULAR SYNCHRONOUS PACING

CI 3.3 L/min/m²
BP 120/70

Figure 7. Physiologic effect on cardiac output and blood pressure by restoration of normal atrioventricular synchrony.

and transmit this signal to the pulse generator which emits an output stimulation pulse through the ventricular lead at an appropriate P-R interval. This, then, creates the most physiologic type of cardiac pacing available in which the ventricular contraction is triggered by a preceding atrial contraction (Fig. 7). This then allows the normal rise and fall in heart rate seen in response to physical or emotional stress.

For patients with undependable atrial mechanisms, the atrial and ventricular leads actively transmit output stimulation impulses to their respective chambers to create atrio ventricular sequential pacing (Fig. 8). This type of pacing has

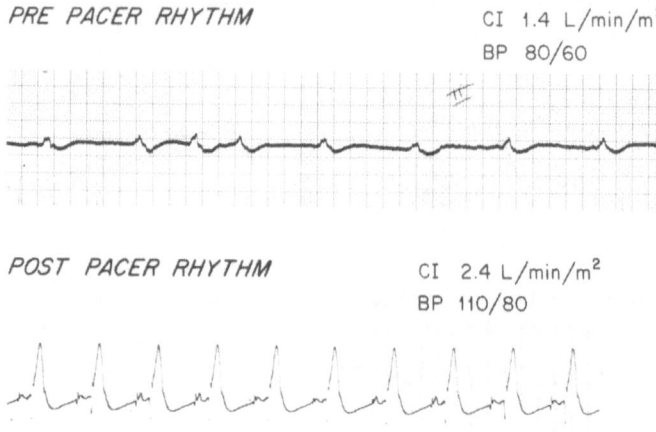

Figure 8. Physiologic effect of atrio-ventricular sequential pacing in a 72 year old male with cardio-myopathy and nodal rhythm.

required somewhat bulky lead systems and pulse generators in the past and has been most commonly used for temporary stimulation of critically ill patients with various types of low output states related to rhythm disorders. Permanently implanted devices have been used on occasion, and will be more commonly employed with the coming availability of smaller programmable units.

Until this point we have discussed the management of bradyarrhythmias alone. In a patient with ventricular or atrial ectopic arrhythmias, some form of cardiac stimulation faster than the customary rate is desirable. From a technical standpoint, ventricular pacing using an externally programmable device is generally the simplest approach. However, these are often patients with serious underlying disorders of cardiac muscle function due to coronary artery disease or primary myocardial disease where cardiac performance may be seriously jeopardized by ventricular stimulation alone. In the setting of overdrive stimulation for suppression of ventricular tachyarrhythmias, pacing alone seldom suffices and some combination of cardiac stimulation combined with drug therapy is usually required (Fig. 9). Stimulation of the heart at rapid rates alone with

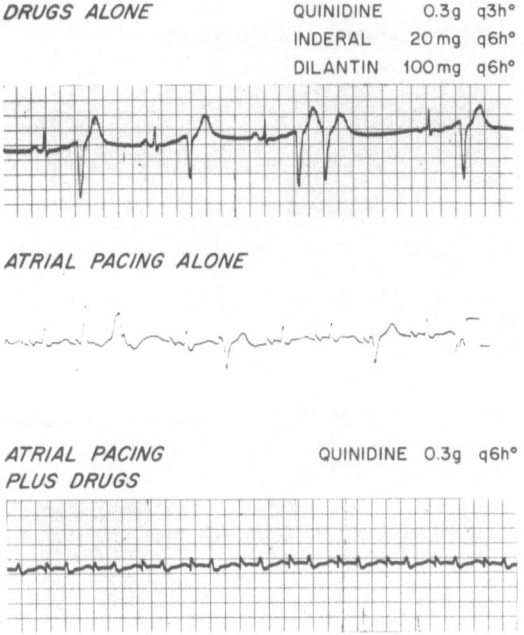

Figure 9. Overdrive suppression of ventricular irritability. Note that pacing alone is ineffective until combined with drug therapy.

drug therapy alters the refractory period of the myocardium and suppresses the emergence of ectopic arrhythmias. The rate necessary to accomplish this goal varies not only from patient to patient, but within the same patient may vary from time to time. For this reason, externally rate programmable units are usually selected.

Whereas the foregoing techniques are designed to suppress the emergence of ectopic activity, the actual conversion once established has recently become possible. This, most commonly entails rapid stimulation of the atrium in patients with various regular supraventricular tachyarrhythmias (Fig. 10). Generally, this is performed in post operative cardiac surgical patients in whom temporary epicardial, atrial (and ventricular) pacing electrodes are left as a matter of routine. With the development of a supraventricular tachycardia, stimulation of the atrium is initiated. This usually requires a stimulation rate of approximately 125% of the underlying atrial arrhythmias. A recent report indicated 100% successful conversion of atrial flutter in 100 consecutive post operative patients in whom this rhythm disorder appeared. A permanent implantable device with similar function is available for patients with difficult-to-control atrial tachyarrhythmias. Here the pacemaker device is activated by the patient through a radio frequency control device.

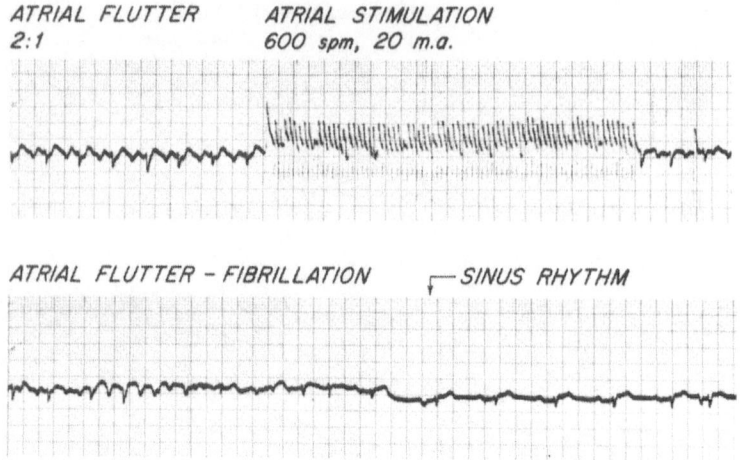

Figure 10. Interruption of atrial tachyarrhythmia through rapid atrial stimulation through post operative transthoracic 'temporary' pacing electrodes.

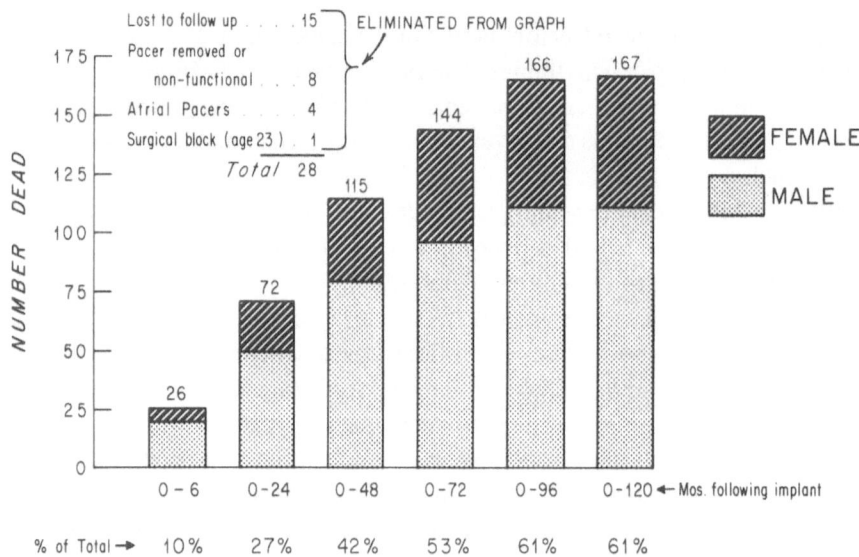

Figure 11. Chronologic followup of the first 272 consecutive patients with transvenous pacemaker systems at the Massachusetts General Hospital from July 1965 until December 1971. Note that 50 % of patients are dead by approximately 5 years – almost entirely of non-pacemaker related causes.

A variety of new devices presently available only for temporary pacing are worthy of mention. The Orthorhythmic pacemaker has been used quite extensively in Europe and more recently in the United States. This device provides the capability of detection of various atrial or ventricular tachyarrhythmias and the initiation of electrical stimulation at a pre-determined, programmed cycle length to interrupt the rhythm disorder. The Threshold Tracking pacemaker introduced by Bowers provides automatic monitoring of beat to beat fluctuations in stimulation threshold with appropriate variation in the output of the circuit. While these and similar innovations remain at the level of research and development, there is little doubt that future implantable systems will have far more sophisticated capabilities than present equipment.

A final word regarding the prognosis of patients undergoing pacemaker insertion is appropriate. Between July 1965 and the present, we have performed 1,000 primary pacemaker insertions at the Massachusetts General Hospital. In a recent review of the first 300 patients done between 1965 and 1971, we find approximately 27% have died within two years and 50% are dead by five to six years (Fig. 11). Thus, it behooves us in considering the appropriate energy source to match it as closely as possible to the projected longevity of the patient. Younger patients without other life threatening diseases may well be selected for nuclear energy sources. On the other hand, those patients whose survival is jeopardized by associated diseases such as diabetes, congestive heart failure or chronic renal disease may be effectively treated with mercury zinc or lithium powered pacers. The clinical features at the time of initial presentation may aid in estimating subsequent survival (Fig. 12). Thus, we find that patients having

ASSOCIATED DISEASES AT TIME OF IMPLANT :

	Death Within 2 yrs	Survival Over 8 yrs
DIABETES	24 of 68 (35%)	6 of 42 (14%)
HYPERTENSION	17 of 68 (25%)	11 of 42 (26%)
CORONARY DISEASE	38 of 68 (56%)	12 of 42 (28%)
CONGESTIVE FAILURE	39 of 68 (59%)	6 of 42 (14%)
PERSISTENT AZOTEMIA	21 of 68 (30%)	2 of 42 (5%)
SENILE DEMENTIA	12 of 68 (17%)	0 of 42 (0%)
MALIGNANCY	7 of 68 (10%)	0 of 42 (0%)

Figure 12. Clinical features of the early mortality and late survival patients depicted in Figure 11. Note the higher incidence of diabetes, coronary disease, congestive failure and impaired renal function in the early mortality group.

shorter prognoses tend to be those with a predominance of left ventricular failure, diabetes, and impaired renal and cerebral function while the late survivors are less frequently afflicted with these disorders at the time of initial pacer implantation.

In summary then, we have reviewed the basic types of cardiac stimulation available to us and made a plea to match the selection of that device to the patient's clinical and physiologic needs. Recognition of the patient's projected survival time based on clinical common sense plays a role in selection of an appropriate energy source. Only the lack of a dependable, stable atrial electrode system holds us back from employing the more sophisticated and more physiologic types of cardiac stimulation such as A-V synchronous or A-V sequential pacing.

Literature

1. Adolph, R.J., Holmes, J.C. and Fukusumi, H., Hemodynamic studies in patients with chronically implanted pacemakers. *Am. Heart J.* 76, 829, 1968.
2. Bevegard, S., Observations on the effect of varying ventricular rate on the circulation at rest and during exercise in two patients with an artificial pacemaker. *Acta Med. Scand.* 172, 615, 1962.
3. Bevegard, S., Jonsson, B., Karlof, I., Lagergren, H. and Sowton, E., Effect of changes in ventricular rate on cardiac output and central pressures at rest and during exercise in patients with artificial pacemakers. *Cardiov. Res.* 1, 21, 1967.
4. Benchimol, A., Li, Y.B., Dimond, R.G., Voth, R.B. and Roland, A.S., Effect of heart rate, exercise and nitroglycerine on the cardiac dynamics in complete heart block. *Circulation* 28, 510, 1963.
5. Benchimol, A., Li, Y.B. and Dimond, E.G., Cardiovascular dynamics in complete heart block at various heart rates: Effect of exercise at a fixed heart rate. *Circulation* 30, 542, 1964.
6. Benchimol, A., Ellis, J.G. and Dimond, E.G., Hemodynamic consequences of atrial and ventricular pacing in patients with normal and abnormal hearts. *Am. J. Med.* 39, 911, 1965.
7. Benchimol, A., Palmero, H., Liggett, M.S. and Dimond, E.G., Influence of digitalization on the contribution of atrial systole to the cardiac dynamics at a fixed ventricular rate. *Circulation* 32, 84, 1965.
8. Benchimol, A., Liggett, M.S., Cardiac haemodynamics during stimulation of the right atrium, right ventricle and left ventricle in normal and abnormal hearts. *Circulation* 33, 933, 1966.
9. Benchimol, A., Cardiac functions during electrical stimulation of the heart. *Am. J. Cardiol.* 17, 27, 1966.
10. Benchimol, A., Wu, T. and Liggett, M.S., Effect of exercise and isoproterenol on the cardiovascular dynamics in complete heart block at various heart rates. *Am. Heart J.* 70, 337, 1965.
11. Brockman, S.K., Cardiodynamics of complete heart block. *Am. J. Cardiol.* 16, 72, 1965.
12. Brockman, S.K., Physiological studies and clinical experience in patients with synchronous and asynchronous pacemakers. *J. Thoracic Cardiovascular Surgery* 51, 864, 1966.
13. Büchner, Ch., Gebhardt, W., Overbeck, W., Amaty Leon, F., Reindell, H., Befunde hämodynamischer Untersuchungen vor und nach Implantation eines elektrischen Schrittmachers. *Thoraxchirurgie* 13, 368, 1965.
14. Carleton, R.A., Sessions, R.W. and Graettinger, J.S., Cardiac pacemakers: Clinical and physiological studies. *Med. N. Amer.* 50, 325, 1966.
15. Escher, D.J.W., Schwedel, J.B., Eisenberg, R., Gitsios, C., Perna, N. and Jamshidi, A., Cardiovascular dynamic responses to artificial pacing in patients in heart block. *Circulation* 24, 928, 1961.

16. Escher, D.J.W., Furman, S. and Solomon, N., Cardiorenal dynamics in paced patients. *Clin. Res.* 16, 228, 1968.
17. Gaal, P.G., Goldberg, S.J. and Linde, L.M., Cardiac output as a function of ventricular rate in a patient with complete heart block. *Circulation* 30, 592, 1964.
18. Gilmore, J.P., Sarnoff, S.J., Mitchell, J.H. and Linden, R.J., Synchronicity of ventricular contractions: Observations comparing hemodynamic effects of atrial and ventricular pacing. *Brit. Heart J.* 25, 299, 1963.
19. Harthorne, J.W., Pohost, G.M., Electrical Therapy of Cardiac Dysrhythmias. *Clinical Cardiovascular Physiology*. Levine, H.J., Eds., Grune and Stratton, New York 853-882, 1976.
20. Harthorne, J.W., Selection of Various Types of Cardiac Pacemakers. *Proceedings of the Pacemaker Colloquium*. Norman, J., and Rickards, A., Eds., Vitatron Medical, Arnhem 1976.
21. Harthorne, J.W. Prognostic Determinants of Late Survival in Patients with Cardiac Pacemakers, *Vth International Symposium on Cardiac Pacing, Tokyo 1976*. Excerpta Medica, Amsterdam 1977.
22. Haupt, G.J., Myers, R.N., Daly, J.W. and Birkhead, N.C., Implanted cardiac pacemakers of variable frequency. *JAMA* 185, 87, 1963.
23. Humphries, J.O., Hinman, E.J., Bernstein, L. and Walker, W.G., Effect of artificial pacing of the heart on cardiac and renal function. *Circulation* 36, 717, 1967.
24. Judge, R.D., Wilson, W.S. and Siegel, J.H., Hemodynamic studies in patients with implanted cardiac pacemakers. *New Eng. J. Med.* 270, 1391, 1964.
25. Kastor, J.A., DeSanctis, R.W., Leinbach, R.C., Harthorne, J.W. and Wolfson, I.N., Long-term pervenous atrial pacing. *Circulation* 40, 535, 1969.
26. Kosowsky, B.D., Stein, E., Lau, S.H., Lister, J.W., Haft, J. and Damato, A.N., A comparison of the hemodynamic effects of tachycardia produced by atrial pacing and atropine. *Am Heart J.* 72, 594, 1966.
27. Kreuzer, H., Bostroem, B., Effert, S., Sykosch, J., Anderung des Herzvolumens bei Patienten mit totalem AV-Block unter dem Einfluss verschiedener Schrittmacherfrequenzen. *Verhandlg. Dtsch. Ges. Kreislaufforschung.* 30, 236, 1944.
28. Leinbach, R.C., Chamberlain, D.A., Kastor, J.A., Harthorne, J.W. and Sanders, C.A., A comparison of the hemodynamic effects of ventricular and sequential atrioventricular pacing in patients with heart block. *Am. Heart J.* 78, 502, 1969.
29. Leonard, J., Kroetz, F., Shaver, J., Taguchi, J. and Laneve, S., The timing of atrial systole as a determinate of left ventricular stoke volume. *Clin. Res.* 12, 55, 1964.
30. Levinson, D.C., Gunther, L., Meehan, J.P. Jr., Griffith, G.C. and Spritzler, R.J., Hemodynamic studies in five patients with heart block and slow ventricular rates. *Circulation* 12, 739, 1955.
31. Levinson, D.C., Shubin, H., Gunther, L. and Meehan, J.P., Hemodynamic findings in heart block with slow ventricular rates. *Am. J. Cardiol.* 4, 440, 1959.
32. Lister, J.W., Stein, E., Kosowsky, B.D. and Damato, A.N., Effects of pacemaker site on cardiac output and ventricular activation in dogs with complete heart block. *Am. J. Cardiol.* 14, 494, 1964.
33. Martin, R.H., Cobb, L.A., Lau, S.H. and Samson, W.E., Impaired cardiac function during ventricular pacing in man. *Clin. Res.* 13, 122, 1965.
34. Muller, O.F. and Bellet, S., Treatment of intractable heart failure in the presence of complete atrioventricular heart block by the use of the internal cardiac pacemaker. *New Eng. J. Med.* 265, 768, 1961.
35. McGregor, M. and Klassen, G.A., Observations on the effect of heart rate on cardiac output in patients with complete heart block at rest and during exercise. *Circ. Res.* (Suppl. 2) 14-15, 215, 1964.
36. McNally, E.M. and Benchimol, A., Medical and physiological considerations in the use of artificial pacing. II. *Am. Heart J.* 75, 679, 1968.
37. Nager, F., Buhlmann, A., Schaub, F., Schmid, J.R., Hämodynamische Befunde bei Patienten mit implantiertem elektrischen Schrittmacher. *Cardiologia* 48, 412, 1966.
38. Pippig, L., Schmitt, W., Gattenlöhner, W., Buck, R., Kardiovaskuläre Dynamik in Abhängigkeit von Schrittmacherinduzierten Herzfrequenzveränderungen bei Patienten mit totalem AV-Block. *Verhandlg. Deutsch. Ges. Inn. Med.* 73, 572, 1967.

39. Ross, J., Linhart, J.W. and Braunwald, E., Effects of changing heart rate in man by electrical stimulation of the right atrium: Studies at rest, during exercise, and with isoproterenol. *Circulation* 32, 549, 1965.

40. Ross, J., Linhart, J.W. and Braunwald, E., Effects of changing heart rate in man by electrical stimulation of the right atrium: Studies at rest during exercise, and with isoproterenol. *Circulation* 32, 549, 1965.

41. Resnekov, L., Sowton, E., Lord, P. and Norman, J., Haemodynamic and clinical effects of paired stimulation of the heart. *Brit. Heart J.* 28, 622, 1966.

42. Samet, P., Jacobs, W., Bernstein, W.H. and Shane, R., Hemodynamic sequelae of idioventricular pacemaking in complete heart block. *Am. J. Cardiol.* 11, 594, 1963.

43. Samet, P., Bernstein, W.H., Nathan, D.A. and Lopez, A., Atrial contribution to cardiac output in complete heart block. *Am. J. Cardiol.* 16, 1, 1965.

44. Samet, P., Castillo, C. and Bernstein, W.H., Hemodynamic consequences of atrial and ventricular pacing in subjects with normal hearts. *Am. J. Cardiol.* 18, 522, 1966.

45. Segel, N., Hudson, W.A., Harris, P. and Bishop, J.M., The circulatory effects of electrically induced changes in ventricular rate at rest and during exercise in complete heart block. *J. Clin. Invest.* 43, 1541, 1964.

46. Sowton, E., The relationship between maximal oxygen uptake and heart rate in patients treated with artificial pacemakers. *Cardiologia* 50, 15, 1967.

47. Sowton, E., Hemodynamic studies in patients with artificial pacemakers. *Brit. Heart J.* 26, 737, 1964.

48. Sowton, E., Thorburn, C., Roy, P., Hemodynamic changes during cardiac pacing. *Proceedings IVth International Symposium on Cardiac Pacing. Groningen, 1973.* Royal Van Gorcum, Assen 24, 1974.

49. Stack, M.F., Rader, B., Sobol, B.J., Farber, S.J. and Eichna, L.W., Cardiovascular hemodynamic functions in complete heart block and the effect of isopropylnorepinephrine. *Circulation* 17, 526, 1958.

50. Stein, E., Damato, A.N., Kosowsky, B.D., Lau, S.H. and Lister, J.W., Cardiovascular responses to alternations in heart rate above and below the sinus rate. *Am. J. Cardiol.* 17, 140, 1966.

51. Stephenson, S.E. and Brockman, S.K., P-wave synchrony. *Ann. N.Y. Acad. Sci.* 111, 907, 1964.

52. Willman, V.L., Howard, H., Riberi, A., Cooper, T. and Hanlon, C.R., Surgical heart block: Influence of electrical pacing, cardiotonic drugs and body temperature. *Arch. Surg.* 83, 496, 1961.

53. Zir, L.M., DeSanctis, R.W. and Harthorne, J.W., Diagnostic Uses of Electrical Pacing, *Diagnostic Methods in Cardiology*, 401-414, 1975.

ELECTRODE DESIGN AND NEW DEVELOPMENTS

HILBERT J. TH. THALEN, M.D.

Introduction

When considering electrodes, one must judge the complete stimulation system. The system is a complex one. It involves electronics, power sources, packaging and is concerned with conduction from the pacemaker to the heart and the electrode interface within the heart muscle. This last subject will be discussed here. In these various areas, a lot of things have happened. In the past, there has been the Mallory battery which is being replaced gradually with the new one, the lithium cell. There is also a changeover in the circuitry from standard components to integrated circuits. The use of integrated circuits and newer energy sources is directed at one goal, to make the pacemaker longer lasting. Longer lasting pacemakers have to be packaged nicely, otherwise the body fluid will enter into it. This complete system of energy source, circuitry, and packaging is very successful now. This would not be worthwhile if it was combined with a very poor electrode. It is the combination of the improvement in electrodes and the other improvements also discussed at this meeting that has brought pacing to the stage of development where a lifetime pacemaker for every patient has almost been reached.

Electrode types

When we talk about electrodes, we have to discuss what we are talking about. The electrode is defined as the uninsulated termination of a lead from a pulse generator which is in direct contact with the heart. We are speaking about the interface between the lead and the heart. The location where you can implant electrodes is variable. The skin electrode applied by Zoll has already been mentioned. But this electrode and the esophageal electrode, also applied in the early days of pacing and now sometimes used for emergency pacing have been abolished mostly because of their indirect contact with the heart that entailed adverse effects during stimulation. A high energy is also needed for effective cardiac stimulation. Epicardial electrodes are electrodes that are placed on the epicar-

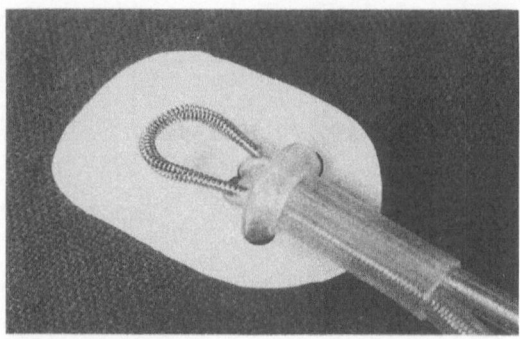

Figure 1. Epicardial loop electrode (Devices).

dium like the disc electrode applied by Elmqvist and Senning or the epicardial loop electrode used by Davis in England (Fig. 1). They don't give too much tissue reaction, but the threshold is not stable enough because of the electrode location. The myocardial or intramural electrodes, like the suture or pin electrode, are implanted into the myocardium. The suture electrode showed a lot of breakages of its wire. It's now used in post operative cases where one has to stimulate the heart only for about eight to ten days. The rigid pin electrode caused a lot of tissue reaction and was also unsuitable. Two intramural electrode designs have

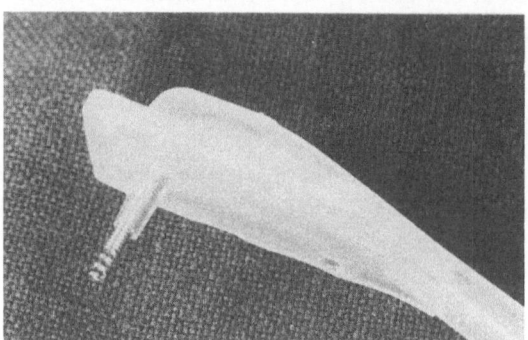

Figure 2. Myocardial coil electrode (Medtronic).

been accepted: the helical pin shaped electrode (Fig. 2) and the loop electrode (Fig. 3). The idea of these electrodes is that you implant them in the epicardium, and they get accepted by the heart. Tissue grows through the helical wire or the loop, embedding the electrode in the heart tissue resulting in less tissue reaction and a nice stimulation threshold. Another intramural electrode developed in recent years is the corkscrew electrode (Fig. 4). This type of electrode has made intramural electrodes a little bit more popular since the introduction of the transvenous or endocardial electrodes that stimulate the heart at the endocardium.

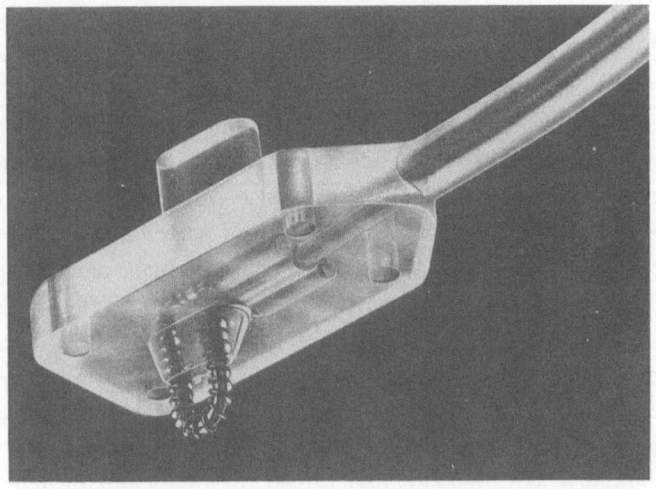

Figure 3. Myocardial loop electrode (Vitatron).

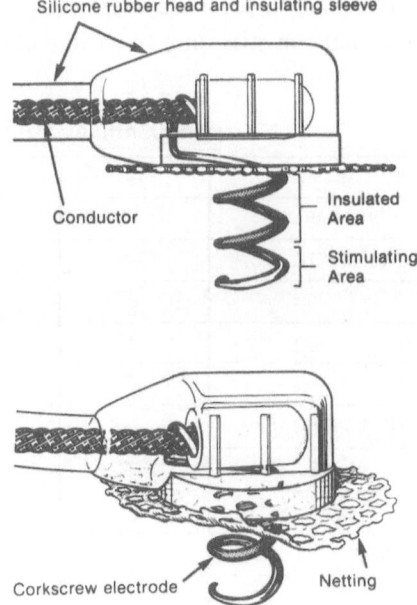

Figure 4. Myocardial corkscrew electrode (Medtronic).

At the Tokyo World Symposium in March 1976 there was a worldwide report of 15,000 electrodes implanted in 1975. Of these 15,000, 93.4% were of the transvenous type and 6.6% of the intramural. Why is transvenous popular? Various points have to be considered (Fig. 5). This is a little bit controversial, but most physicians believe that the ease of inserting an endocardial electrode is a distinct advantage and thus prefer the transvenous route. Some surgeons think the ease of inserting a myocardial electrode is about the same as an endocardial system. The stability of a myocardial electrode is a big point to take advantage of especially the early stability and with it goes also a stable threshold, whereas transvenous endocardial electrodes have a certain percentage of dislocations. Use of the epicardial screw tip lead system has the advantage of easier insertion through a sub-xiphoid incision in contrast to the other epicardial lead systems which require a thoracotomy to permit suture fixation. However, the endocardial electrode has a lot of advantages. The morbidity and mortality post operatively is a little bit lower, although this is also acceptable with myocardial implants in experienced centers, but what is very important is the greater patient's acceptance. Most patients prefer local anesthesia and it is much easier and also less dangerous. Another advantage is the ease of removal, especially in the case of an infected electrode which is much easier with an endocardial electrode whereas with a myocardial electrode another thoracotomy is necessary. The post operative hospital stay is a little bit variable. We now have our patients staying in the hospital about five to seven days after a primary endocardial implantation. It also seems that convalescence from an endocardial implant is

	ENDOCARDIAL	MYOCARDIAL
EASE OF INSERTION	=	=
STABILITY OF POSITION •EARLY		√
•LATE	=	=
P.O. MORBIDITY	√	
P.O MORTALITY	√	
PATIENT ACCEPTANCE	√	
THRESHOLD STABILITY • SHORT TERM		√
• LONG TERM	=	=
EASE OF REMOVAL	√	
POST-OP. HOSPITAL STAY	√	
OVERALL COST	√	
FLEXIBILITY	√	
	√	

Figure 5. Advantages and Disadvantages of endocardial vs. myocardial electrodes (courtesy of Dr. Victor Parsonnet).

shorter than with a myocardial one. These facts have made the transvenous endocardial electrode type the most commonly selected electrode.

Bipolar vs. monopolar electrodes

Another topic which must be discussed when one considers electrodes is the controversy, (more pronounced in the United States than in Europe) between bipolar and monopolar electrodes. Monopolar electrodes have been popular in Europe from the beginning (Fig. 6). In the United States their acceptance has taken more time. First of all, there is only one electrode in contract with the heart. This means that with transvenous electrodes you do not have to bother about the contact of the second one. Of course there also is a disadvantage of having only one electrode within the heart. When this electrode breaks you have to repair or change the electrode, whereas with a bipolar system, the defective electrode can be used as an indifferent electrode for a modified monopolar system, which uses the intact electrode of the bipolar system for the stimulation electrode. What's very important, however, with the monopolar system is the

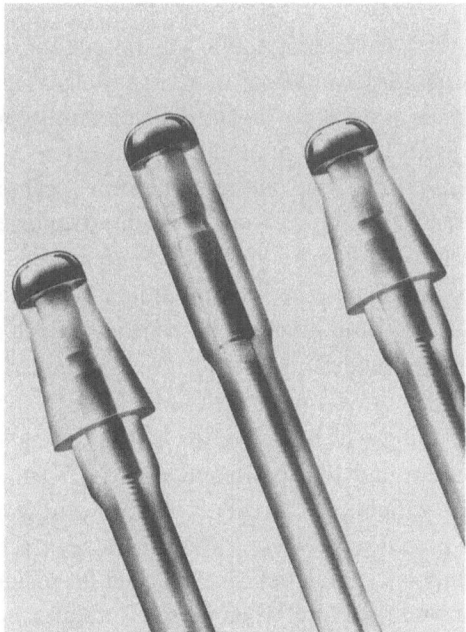

Figure 6. Endocardial monopolar transvenous electrodes with surface areas of approximately 24 mm.

free choice of the indifferent electrode. A large surface electrode can be selected, which has a low resistance and enables one to stimulate the heart with a low voltage. Another important feature is that the current density of the large indifferent electrodes is minimized preventing problems of electrolysis. This also makes the choice of the electrode material easier. Stainless steel or Titanium are commonly used for this indifferent electrode that is usually a plate attached to the pacemaker itself or comprises the encapsulation of the pacemaker circuitry and epoxy batteries. The lead for a monopolar electrode only needs one wire. That makes it simple and more flexible, and only one connecting attachment to the generator is necessary. During subsequent pacemaker patient follow-up, a large dipole results, and this provides an easier check of the pacemaker system. Another important feature is that monopolar stimulation seems to present lower cardiac vulnerability to competition with fewer ventricular tachycardias or even ventricular fibrillation. It has been demonstrated that these phenomena, although rather rare, are more commonly seen with bipolar stimulation probably because of cardiac stimulation at the positive electrode or the anode in the vulnerable phase. The anodal threshold in that phase especially during the first post implant period is lower than the cathodal or negative one. Another feature of monopolar pacing is that with one electrode in the heart and the other outside, the current has to go through the myocardium whereas with an endocardial bipolar system, it can go partly through the blood, reducing maximum current in the myocardium.

There is controversy concerning the R-wave signal for detection. It appears that bipolar leads have a lower signal than monopolar. This is still not proven and various publications are reporting conflicting results. We believe from our data that the R-wave is larger in monopolar stimulation.

There are of course some disadvantages when one speaks about a monopolar system in comparison to a bipolar one. The disadvantage is that muscle interference may occur with demand monopolar pacemakers. When a pacemaker is located in the pectoral area, the pectoral muscle can generate myopotentials which are picked up by the indifferent electrode and which can block the pacemaker. With the newer models, these effects are minimized or prevented completely by the pacemaker reverting to the fixed rate mode and this is seldom seen anymore. Another thing which may occur is that during stimulation, muscle contractions occur around the indifferent electrode. Sometimes this can be bothersome for the patient, but usually if you are careful at implantation the pacemaker can be placed somewhere where muscle contractions do not occur.

In general, monopolar stimulation, has reached far greater acceptance than bipolar stimulation and therefore, when we speak about a pacemaker electrode today, we usually have to deal with an endocardial monopolar electrode.

What do we expect from this pacemaker electrode? We expect three things. We expect *stable contact with the heart.* We expect an *efficient stimulation with low energy consumption* and for the demand pacemaker, we expect also *reliable detection of myocardial activity.*

Electrode fixation

How do we get stable contact with the heart? When you make a stiff electrode and electrode wire, introduction into the right ventricle and contact with the endocardium could be improved but you will have a great possibility of penetration and even perforation of the myocardium. In many cases of perforation cardiac stimulation is maintained because the pericardium pushes the electrode against the epicardium. Hiccups caused by stimulation of the phrenic nerve or the diaphragm itself and especially exit blocks because of the unreliable electrode position are early warnings of a perforation that is usually difficult to diagnose by X-ray because of the superimposition of the left ventricle. Usually not much of a tamponade is found because the catheter blocks the canal through the myocardium. However, the longterm result remains insecure and therefore stiff catheters do not bring a solution to catheter dislocation but create more difficulties. Since dislocation of the transvenous electrodes is still reported in experienced clinics in 3-9% of cases, techniques of fixing the electrode in the right ventricle, especially for the first post implant period, have been investigated. Some of the principles of fixation will be discussed. One method comes from Germany from the group of Vogel and Schaldach (Fig. 7). After introduction of the electrode, an inner tip is pushed and consists of a single wire 'umbrella frame' which springs out to anchor itself between the trabecular muscles. Withdrawal of this catheter for repositioning, e.g. in the case of a high stimulation threshold, seems very difficult because tissue fixes itself in and around the tip and prevents

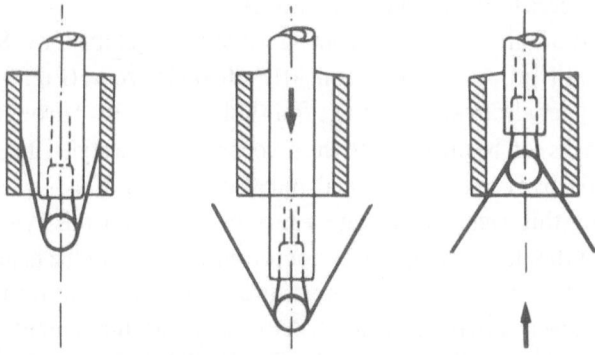

Figure 7. Biotronik hooking electrode after Vogel et al.

reversal of the mechanism in the tip of the electrode. In some cases this electrode has also been used for atrial sensing and stimulation. Since its introduction in 1970, it has not gained wide acceptance. The same holds for a modification by Irnich intended originally for atrial stimulation (Fig. 8). This electrode, of which about 1000 have been implanted, fixes itself by two metal wires that advance antegrade and penetrate the myocardium rather than retrograde as with the previous electrode.

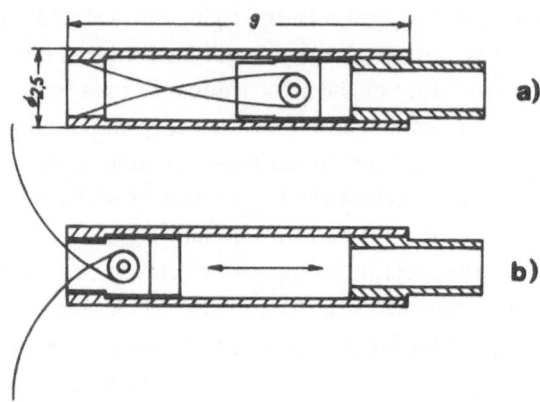

Figure 8. Biotronik hooking electrode after Irnich.

Both electrodes have similar disadvantages. Fixation occurs at the same point where they stimulate. Fixation causes tissue reaction and tissue reaction influences the stimulation threshold in a negative way. The Vogel type of electrode has a large low ohmic tip and the long term threshold sometimes increases to such a value that normal pacemakers are unable to stimulate the heart. The Irnich electrode has a smaller surface. Long term results are not reported in sufficient numbers to draw final conclusions.

Another solution came also from Germany, developed by Schmidt and modified by our group, the Vitatron MIP-2000 electrode (Fig. 9). This is an ordinary catheter electrode which has four holes in the tip. Through these holes four nylon barbs can be pushed into the myocardium by a stylet. The angle under which these barbs arise is very critical and also the kind of nylon used is important. By using this system, one gets a nice fixation with the nylon barbs and stimulation at the electrode tip. I was not too enthusiastic in the beginning about this electrode, but there have been implants of over 4,000. This means that some people do very well with this approach. A further idea which comes from Sweden is the Siemens Elema balloon electrode (Fig. 10). This provides for the inflation of a small balloon near the tip. It is suggested that the balloon fixes the electrode

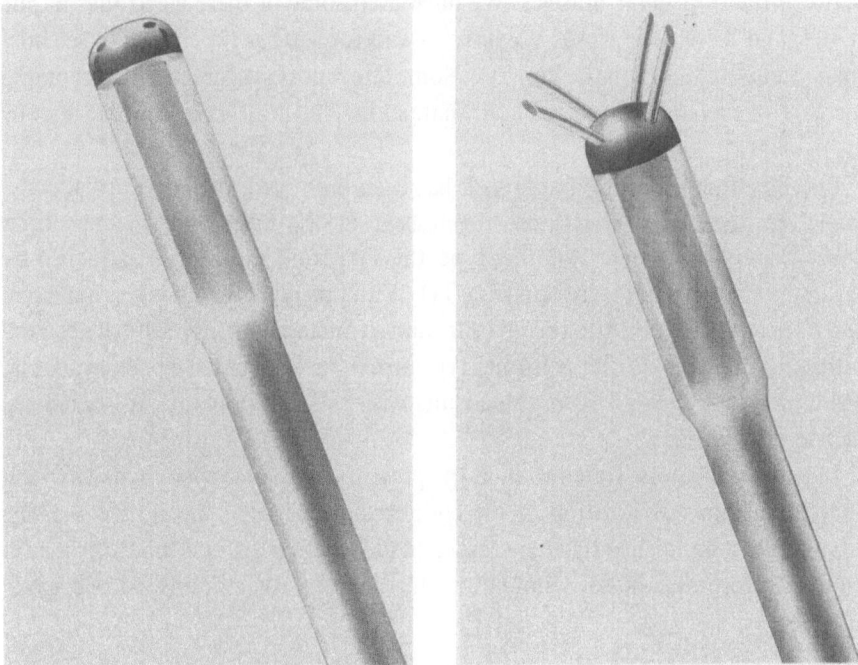

Figure 9. Vitatron MIP 2000 electrode with barbs retracted (panel A) and extended (panel B) after Schmidt.

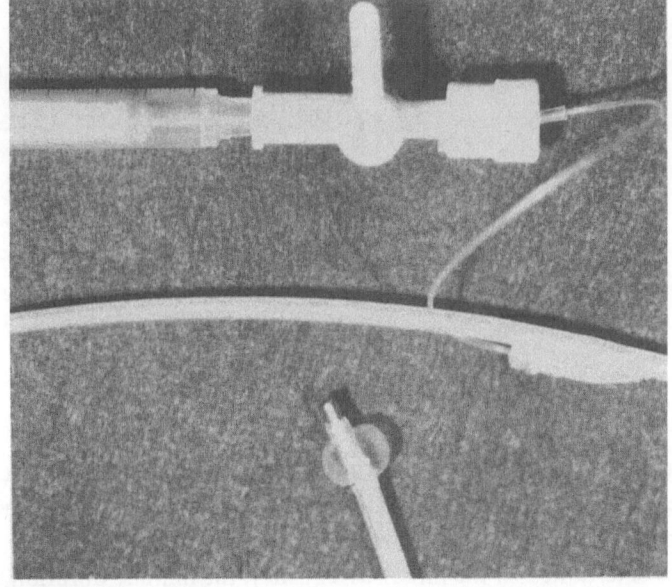

Figure 10. Siemens-Elema balloon electrode.

between the trabecular muscles. We have used some of these electrodes in our center, and it seems to work. We have to wait for further experience to see how this system functions on the long run. Some late reports suggest an unacceptable increase of the stimulation treshold that, so far, has not been recorded by our group.

Recently another fixation approach has been promoted: the endocardial cork-screw electrode. The type most reminiscent of the epicardial one has been developed by Medtronic. Another type, the Vitatron Helifix is also attached by turning a kind of a corkscrewtip (Fig. 11). With this type, the tip is less agressive and does not penetrate into the myocardium so much but turns itself between the trabecular muscles. With the former type no extensive data have been available. The latter type showed favorable results with the first implants; a limited experience, however.

In general it can be stated that, at the present time, some systems exist which enable an improved fixation of the endocardial electrode. In most cases, the advantage is diminished by an increased tissue reaction around the electrode tip and therefore increased stimulation threshold with diminished electrode efficiency.

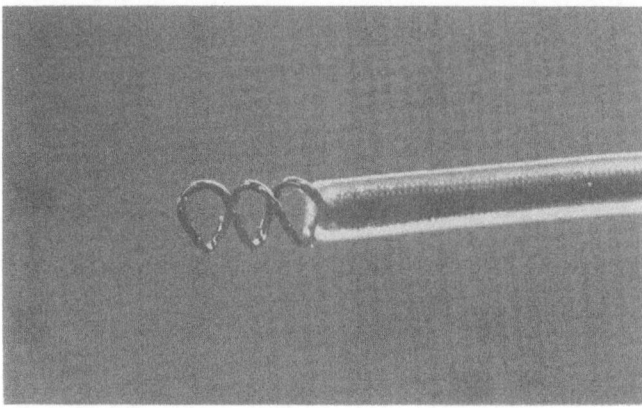

Figure 11. Vitatron Helifix electrode after Babotai et al.

Efficiency of the electrode systems

Apart from fixation of the electrode within the heart, we have to discuss the efficiency of an electrode, especially when we are considering lifetime pacemaker systems. Therefore, we must discuss the energy needed for cardiac stimulation. That is determined by the impulse frequency, the impulse duration, the stimulation threshold and the safety margin. The electrode can affect this stimulation threshold and of course, allied to it, the safety margin.

What determines the stimulation threshold? It's an interaction between the myocardium with the electrode and the impulse that's applied to the heart. The *state of the myocardium* is important for the stimulation threshold. If you have a myocardium with much fibrous tissue, it will not be easy to find a low stimulation threshold. Electrolytes, for instance potassium, and hormones like glucocorticosteroids influence the stimulation threshold. Some drugs such as prednisone also have an influence on the stimulation threshold. Potassium is important in cases of diabetics where you might have a high cellular influx and outflux of potassium when you give these patients insulin. These changes in the stimulation threshold are intrinsic to the patient. We have to recognize and accept them. They influence the safety margin of the pacemaker systems. With the electrode, we can influence the stimulation threshold. Let's first look at the *pacemaker impulse*. When we look at the impulse polarity, we know, that cathodal or negative stimulation has the lowest threshold. This is an accepted fact now and therefore all impulses given to the heart are negative and the indifferent electrode is connected to the positive pole of the pacemaker system. We also know that when we decrease the pulse width, we get an increase of stimulation threshold. Some years ago we were all using pacers with impulse durations of 2 milliseconds, but now we are moving to 1.0, 0.5, and even 0.25 milliseconds. At the present time, we stimulate negative with as small a pulse width as possible. This pulse width depends upon the stimulation threshold that is largely influenced by the stimulation electrode. The surface area of the electrode is very critical. The fact that small electrodes provide lower stimulation thresholds than those with large surface areas has already been known from the beginnings of cardiac stimulation but its consequences have only been recognized during recent years. Originally we used electrodes with a surface area of about 50 mm²; about 8-10 years ago we began using electrodes with areas of 20-28 mm² until two or three years ago when the surface area was reduced to 12 or 10 mm². At present we have some electrodes like the Vitatron LOE and Cordis ball tip that are 8 mm² and even now there are some experimental electrodes with a 5 mm² surface area. How far should we go down in surface area to get the lowest stimulation threshold, and is there an optimal surface area?When you look at the relation between current thresholds and electrode, the stimulation threshold could be extrapolated until about 0. Well this is nonsense of course, but you could get close to that level when you have a very small surface area. Recent studies seem to indicate that extrapolation is justified until a radius of about 0.3 mm. Beyond that level no further decrease of stimulation threshold can be demonstrated. This is most probably due to the area of the critical cell mass to be depolarized for a propagated depolarization wave across the whole heart.

We should not look only at the current threshold, however, but also to voltage threshold. The voltage is the current multiplied by the resistance. When we decrease the surface area of an electrode, we increase the resistance of the electrode system. At a certain point with decreasing surface area the benefit of the smaller current threshold is over shadowed by the increase of the resistance. This means that when we look at the voltage threshold, we get a U-shaped curve and we never reach a 0 level. The minimal value of the voltage threshold can be calculated as has been done by Irnich. With this calculation, we have also to keep in mind the tissue reaction around the electrode. This fibrous tissue can conduct the impulse without difficulty and has about the same resistance as myocardial tissue but increases the effective electrode area. The calculation demonstrates that the voltage reaches its minimum when the radius of that electrode is as large as the density of the tissue reaction around it. If we are able to find out the tissue reaction around the electrode, we know roughly what the radius of that electrode should be. Evaluation and calculation of stimulation threshold with electrodes with known surface areas show this to be roughly 1 mm. We therefore developed an electrode with a radius of 1 mm (Fig. 12). This low output electrode (LOE)

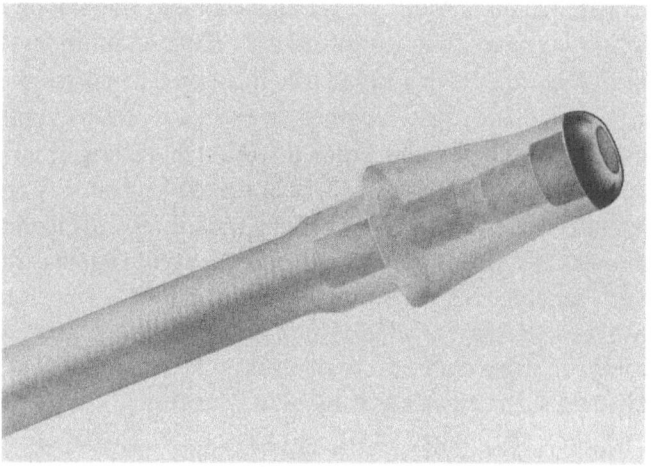

Figure 12. Endocardial transvenous low output electrode (Vitatron LOE).

had a surface area of about 7.6 mm². As only the electrode area with a high current density was selected to conduct the impulse, the electrode was designed in a ring shape. Evaluation in four clinics gave promising results. The data of Kleinert who participated with the Hamburg-Harburg Clinics in the evaluation and who sometimes implants in two steps are shown in the figure (Fig. 13). The data pertain to 27 implants using Medtronic electrodes with small surface areas and the Vitatron LOE. These data demonstrate that the current threshold of the Vitatron LOE is lower than with the Medtronic small surface electrode ($\pm$ 12 mm²). The current threshold reaches a maximum between the ninth and the tenth day and then goes down. The resistance, however, of the LOE, because of its small surface is higher. This means that the difference between the voltage thresholds is less than it is for the current. However, the current (multiplied by

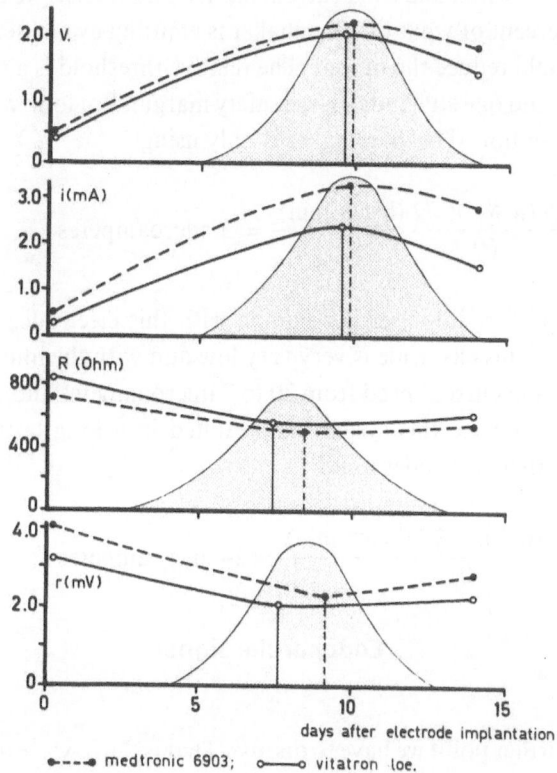

Figure 13. Variation in various parameters during 15 days after implantation of seven transvenous Medtronic Model # 6903 (11 mm²) and nine transvenous Vitatron LOE (8 mm²) electrodes.

time is charge) is what is drained from the batteries and determines the pacemaker's lifetime. In this respect the electrode only needs a low output and also diminishes the battery drain because of its higher resistance and has therefore promising features regarding pacemaker life expectancy. Also interesting when you look at the figure is that when you follow the resistance, you see that this resistance also reaches a minimal level which occurs about the seventh day. And just at that seventh day also the detected R-wave reaches its minimal. We found that at the seventh or eighth day from these data, the R-wave is about 70-75% of the R-wave at implant and thereafter increases a bit. These data indicate that when you implant pacers, you will reach, on the average, your highest

threshold at about the tenth day and the lowest R-wave at about the seventh. So
when lead performance, not regarding minor or major dislocations, is satisfactory after fourteen days, it will be adequate for longer lasting systems. After
observing this early data, we implanted more LOE electrodes and were able to
make external stimulation threshold measurements. We found that with a 1
millisecond pulse width and 8 ma current limited pacemaker, we had a threshold
of about 30 percent of what the pacemaker is emitting even after 600 days. We
thought we could reduce the output. The relative threshold is a little bit higher,
not too much, and one still finds a large safety margin. But look what is gained in
current consumption. This pacemaker is only using:

$$\frac{0.5 \ (\text{msec}) \times 5 \ (\text{mA}) \times 72 \ (\text{beats/min})}{60} = 3 \ \text{microamperes}$$

at a frequency of 72 impulses per minute with this electrode. So the current
consumption of this electrode is very very low and with the improved circuitry
that went down in current need from 30 to 3 microamperes and with the longer
lasting energy sources, this system has resulted in a long lasting pacemaker
whereas the earlier electrodes used:

$$\frac{2 \ (\text{msec}) \times 10 \ (\text{mA}) \times 72 \ (\text{beats/min})}{60} = 24 \ \text{microamperes}$$

Endocardial signal

There is one further point we have to discuss. That is the R-wave detection where
two parameters are important: the amplitude and the intrinsic frequency. R-
wave detection depends on a lot of things. It's of course dependent on the state of
the myocardium. When you have right ventricular hypertrophy, you will find a
larger R-wave. It can be as much as 40 or 50 percent higher than with a normal
heart. Infarction also is very important. It causes sometimes a lower R-wave
amplitude, but what is more important is that it provides, during the acute phase,
and R-wave with an even lower frequency content. The frequency of the heart
rate itself is also very important. When you increase the frequency, you may see
increases in R-wave of over 50 percent. Extracardiac phenomena influence also
the detected R-wave. Respiration is very important. Respiration and frequency
probably have one underlying physiological phenomenon in common. That is
the filling status of the ventricle.

In this presentation, the influence of the electrode system should be considered. We know that myocardial electrodes give a higher R-wave than endocar-

dial ones. Monopolar electrode systems most probably give a higher signals than bipolar electrode systems. But what's very important is the ratio between the resistance of the electrode system and the resistance of the pacemaker circuit. When you have an electrode with a resistance of 1,000 ohms and the resistance of the electronic pacemaker circuitry is also 1,000 ohms, the pacemaker will see only $\frac{1}{2}$ of the R-wave which appears at the tip of the electrode. However, when the electrode has a resistance of 1,000 and the circuitry has a resistance of about 20-40,000 ohms then about all of the R-waves will be sensed by the circuit and will be seen by the pacemaker. With the small area of electrodes with resistances between 800-1200 ohms in comparison to the 200-300 ohms of the earlier larger surface types, this has presented some problems with certain pacemaker models that had internal resistances of 2-3000 ohms. In the new pacemaker types, internal resistances of 20-40,000 ohms are applied and this problem has almost been completely overcome.

Conclusion

In conclusion, we will show you a survey (Fig. 14) that demonstrates what we have gained with the various steps, part of which will be discussed in subsequent presentations. The first improvement made concerned electrodes. We reduced the surface area for cardiac stimulation. And by these smaller electrodes, the lifetime of the pacemakers was increased from about two years to about three years. Then better batteries were used, the modified Mallory battery, and in-

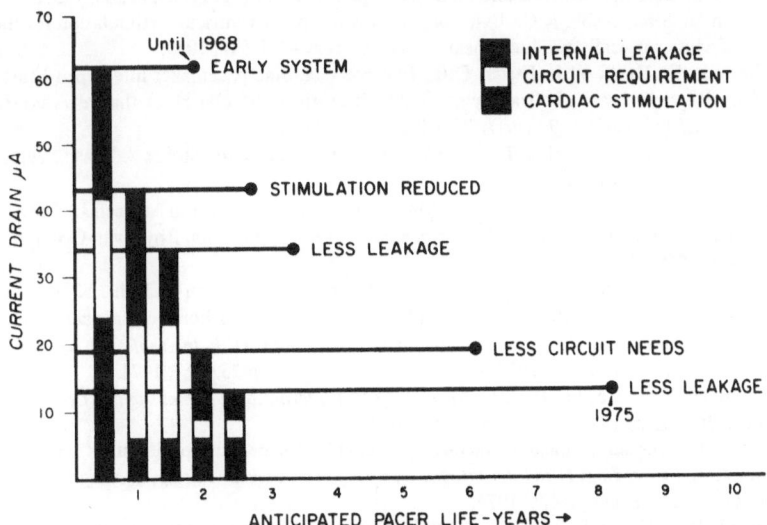

Figure 14. Influence of improvements in battery design, electronic circuit and electrode design (cardiac stimulation) on pacemaker life time. The influence of lithium batteries is not included.

creased it further to more than three years. And then we get big improvements in circuitry, the lower energy consuming circuitry, which extends function to about six years. Further improvements involved low internal battery leakage, and could give pacemakers that go for eight or nine years, and now you can calculate that for some of the lithium units, one can anticipate about twenty years.

However, I mentioned in my earlier remarks to be humble. We have to wait to see what physiology does when physics starts to calculate. The electrode problem is far from solved completely. The electrode lead – redundancy systems – needs attention and the ideal atrial electrode – if it exists at all – still has to be found. There will be a lot of further electrode discussions at this meeting and at other meetings in the future, but some of the electrode problems have been solved however as this presentation has tried to outline.

Literature

1. Zoll, P.M., Resuscitation of the heart in ventricular standstill by external electric stimulation. *New England J. Med.* 247, 768, 1952.
2. Zoll, P.M., A history of electric cardiac stimulation. *Proceedings IVth International Symposium on Cardiac Pacing, Groningen 1973.* Royal van Gorcum, Assen 4-14, 1974.
3. Shafiroff, B.G.P. and Linder J., Effects of external electric pacemaker stimuli on the human heart. *J. Thorac. Surg.* 33, 544, 1957.
4. Thevenent, A., Hodges, P.D. and Lillehei, C.W., The use of a myocardial electrode inserted percutaneously for control of complete atrioventricular block by an artificial pacemaker. *Diseases of the Chest.* 34, 621, 1958.
5. Weirich, W.L., Gott. V.L. and Lillehei, C.W., The treatment of complete block by the combined use of a myocardial electrode and an artificial pacemaker. *Surg. Forum* 8, 360, 1957.
6. Brockman, S.K., Webb, R.C., Bahnson, H.T., Monopolar ventricular stimulation for the control of acute surgically produced heart block. *Surgery* 44-5, 910, 1958.
7. Olmstedt, F., Kolff, W.J., Essler, D.B., Electronic cardiac pacemaker after open heart operations. Report of case of tetralogy of Fallot with atrioventricular block that reverted to sinus rhythm. *Cleveland Clin. Quarterly* 25, 84, 1958.
8. Furman, S. and Schwedel, J.B., AN intracardiac pacemaker for Stokes-Adams seizures. *New England J. Med.* 261, 943, 1958.
9. Thalen, H.J.Th., Van den Berg, J.W., Homan van der Heide, J.N. and Nieveen J., *The Artificial Cardiac Pacemaker, its history, development and clinical application.* Royal van Gorcum, Assen 125-195, 1969.
10. Homan van der Heide, J.N., Bosma, G.J., Kleine, W.J., Thalen H.J.Th., Nieveen, J. and Bartstra, M., Results with pacemaker implantations. Is the transthoracic approach and implantation of intramural electrode still justified. *Proceedings IVth International Symposium on Cardiac Pacing, Groningen 1973.* Royal Van Gorcum, Assen 253-267, 1974.
11. Watanabe, Y. ed. Cardiac Pacing, *Proceedings Vth International Symposium on Cardiac Pacing, Tokyo 1976.* Excerpta Medica, Amsterdam 1977.
12. Sutton, R., The importance of the endocardial QRS for demand pacing in acute myocardial infarction. *Proceedings IVth International Symposium on Cardiac Pacing, Groningen 1973.* Royal van Gorcum, Assen 421-424, 1974.
13. Kurnik, P.B., Cywinski, J.K., Zir, L.M., Newall, J.B., Harthorne, J.W., Frequency and amplitude analysis of endocardial electrograms, Implications for demand pacemaker design.
14. Weidmann, S., *Elektrophysiologie der Herzmuskelfaser.* Huber, Bern 1956.

15. Cole, K.S., *Membranes, ions and impulses.* Berkley 1968.
16. Thalen, H.J.Th., *Elektroden fur Herzschrittmacher.* In press.
17. Irnich W., *Elektrostimulation des Herzens.* Habilitations schrift, T.H. Aachen 1973.
18. Irnich, W., Considerations in electrode design for permanent pacing. *Proceedings IVth International Symposium on Cardiac Pacing, Groningen, 1973.* Royal Van Gorcum, Assen 269-274, 1974.
19. Lagergren, H. and Westerholm, C.J., Electrodes for cardiac pacing. *Proceedings IVth International Symposium on Cardiac Pacing, Groningen 1973.* Royal Van Gorcum, Assen 235-238, 1974.
20. Thalen, H.J.Th., Stimulation electrodes, Past, Present, Future. *Proceedings of the pacemaker colloquium.* Norman, J. and Rickards, A., eds. Vitatron Medical, Arnhem 1976.
21. Greatbatch, W., Electrochemical polarization of physiological electrodes. *Med. Res. Engrg.* 6, 13, 1967.
22. Furman, S., Personal Communication.
23. Thalen, H.J.Th., Pacemaker Longevity. *Proc. Workshop on Cardiac Pacing.* American College of Cardiology, New York 1973.
24. Preston, Th.A., Anodal stimulation as a cause of pacemaker induced ventricular fibrillation. *Am. Heart J.* 6-3, 366, 1973.
25. Cranefield, P.F., Hoffman, B.F. and Siebens, A.A., Anodal excitation of cardiac muscle. *Am. J. Physiol.* 190-383, 1957.

PACEMAKER ENERGY SOURCES

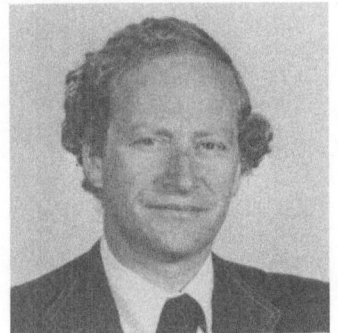

Dr. Josef Cywinski received his master of science degree in electronics at the Warsaw Institute of Technology in 1960 where he specialized in Medical Electronics and Radiation Physics. He later concentrated on Computer Science and Bioengineering and earned his Ph.D. degree in 1967. He emigrated to the United States in 1967 and after several years of basic research at the Universities of Pennsylvania and Missouri, became affiliated with the Massachusetts Institute of Technology and Harvard Medical School. Since 1972 he has been Director of the Department of Medical Engineering at the Massachusetts Genral Hospital. He is the author of many scientific papers in the field of bioengineering research and a member of several international medical and engineering societies.

PACEMAKER ENERGY SOURCES

JOSEF CYWINSKI, PH.D.

Introduction

I would like to begin with the bicentennial theme. 'Power to the people' an appropriate saying, refers to Figure 1. This is a people-powered pacemaker 1932 A.D., and you can imagine standing by the patient's bedside and winding the spring every six minutes. Now we are faced with the same recharging problem except that the time scale is different. Now we have a time span for elective battery replacement of three, six, maybe eight years and some nuclear pacemakers may last over fifteen years. Also the means of powering the pacemaker circuitry are different. Now we use electro-chemical cells, solid state cells, and we use nuclear power to achieve increased pacemaker longevity. There is some laboratory work in progress on other sorts of cells. In this talk I would like to review the choices and the characteristics of a variety of power sources.

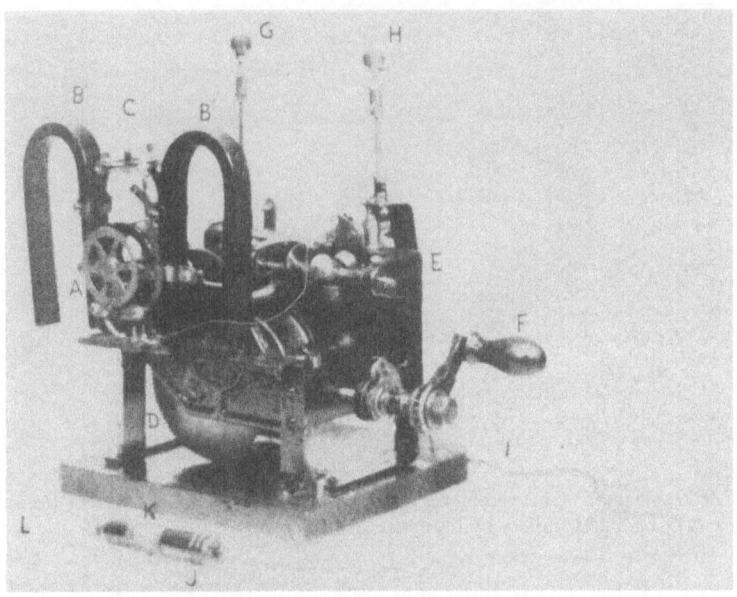

Figure 1. Hyman's 'Artificial Cardiac Pacemaker' (1932).

Chemical cells

Early implantable pacemakers in the United States looked like the one seen in Figure 2 and were powered by a mercury zinc battery inside the generator package. Energy source is obviously a major contributing factor to the pacemaker's longevity. Most of the pacemakers built up to now are closed encapsulated systems, so whatever energy they have contained within the package, they have to live with, and that determines their useful lifetime. Their energy is drained in two ways: by the electronic circuit as outlined by Dr. Thalen and by energy delivered to a pacing electrode. Striking advances have been made in reducing both. Also, the energy source has advanced since the age of the first mercury batteries, and now we have a wide choice of power supplies. The oldest and most venerable is the Ruben mercury cell which is a primary zinc mercuric oxide cell, and interestingly enough, this pacemaker cell is beginning to demonstrate early signs of its obsolescence on the market. I have some figures on sales of pacemakers powered by various power sources. In 1973, 99% of the pacemakers were powered by mercury cells and in 1975 when the total volume of sales of the pacemakers doubled, only 89% by mercury zinc and in 1976, 81%. So the trend for this type of power is downward at the expense of the lithium cells which are gaining the market share. Other cells, like rechargeable cells, are responsible for a very small fraction of the market, only 1%. Well, let's look at mercury cells and see what are the characteristics and advantages which determine that this was the

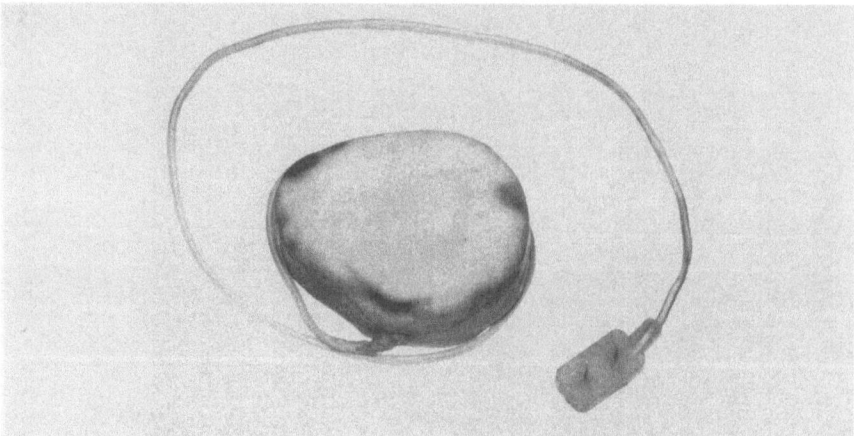

Figure 2. Early Medtronic implantable pacemaker with electrode (1960): contained 10 RM-1 cells and weighed close to one pound (courtesy Keith Fester, Medtronic).

cell of choice at the beginning and why it is fading away now from the market. Fig. 3 depicts the testing results of the improved Rm. 1 Group 2 mercury zinc

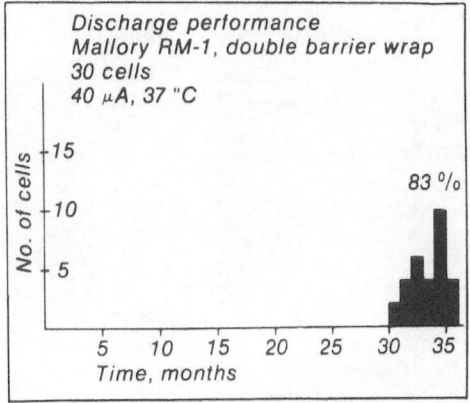

Figure 3. Graph of Rm 1 Group 2 cell depletion (Medtronic).

cell of choice at the beginning and why it is fading away now from the market. Fig. 3 depicts the testing results of the improved Rm. 1 Group 2 mercury zinc cells and shows that cell depletion is clustered around 30 months. Some manufac-

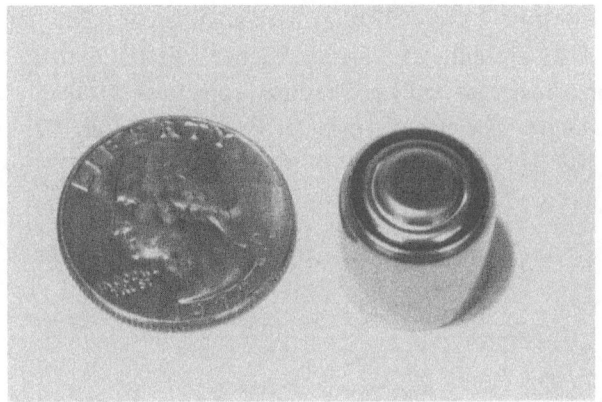

Figure 4. Photograph of Rm 1 mercury zinc cell (courtesy Keith Fester, Medtronic).

turers project that pacemakers powered by improved mercury cells can now survive for sixty months or five years. Figure 4 shows a single cell which is used in pacemaker construction, though usually arranged in series configuration of four or five cells. Figure 5 is a cutaway of the cell which shows the zinc anode and mercuric oxide cathode placed concentrically in a cylindrical container which is made of a stainless steel alloy. In between this anode and cathode, there is electrolyte and depolarizer. The electrolyte is sodium or potassium hydroxide of a strongly corrosive nature and is alkaline. The byproduct of the energy dis-

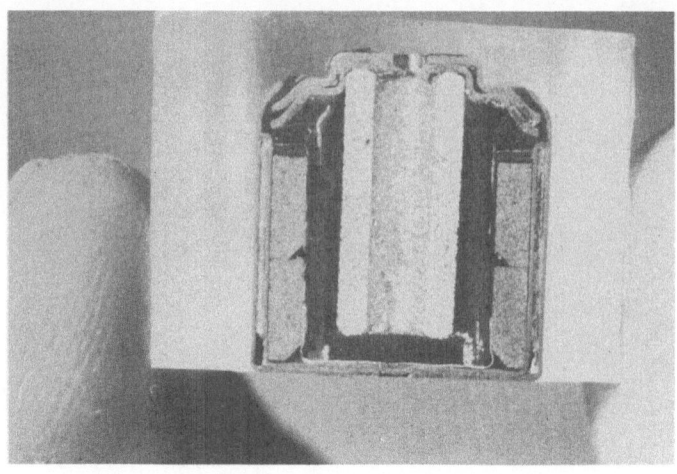

Figure 5. Cutaway of Rm 1 mercury zinc cell (courtesy Keith Fester, Medtronic).

charge of the cell is metallic mercury and since this is a metal can, this can eventually cause a short circuit between the anode and the cathode thus resulting in battery failure. Even though these cells have been made to high reliability standards and with extreme care plus some technological improvements which have been added in 1972 and 1973, they have an inherent failure mode in their construction. They are built of a highly reactive material (zinc and mercury) immersed in a corrosive electrolyte. They are prone to short circuits by metallic deposits of mercury. The improvement of the cell made in 1973 provided a double wrap separator (Figure 6) to prevent the dendrite growth of metallic

Cell Voltage: 1.35v
Rated Capacity: 1.0 Amp-hr.

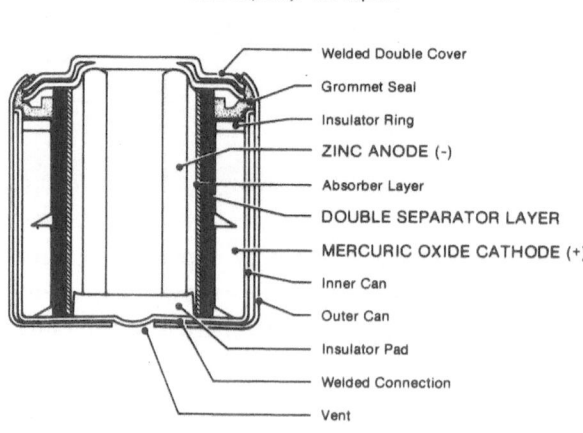

Welded Double Cover
Grommet Seal
Insulator Ring
ZINC ANODE (-)
Absorber Layer
DOUBLE SEPARATOR LAYER
MERCURIC OXIDE CATHODE (+)
Inner Can
Outer Can
Insulator Pad
Welded Connection
Vent

Figure 6. Diagram of 'improved' Rm 1 mercury zinc cell with double-wrap separator (courtesy Keith Fester, Medtronic).

mercury from the outer cylinder into the inner zinc anode. By using this double wrap, manufacturers claimed that it would be much more difficult for dendrite to penetrate the pinholes in the separator and short out the cell. Indeed the longevity of this cell in pacemakers is much better.

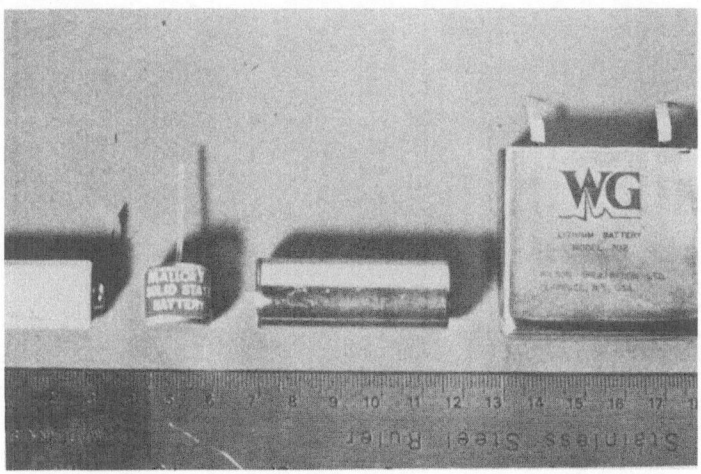

Figure 7. Different types of lithium cells: (a) Gould (b) Mallory (c) General Telephone and Electronics (d) Greatbatch.

Lithium cells (Figure 7) came on the market in 1973 and were introduced by Wilson Greatbatch who started work on them in 1970, and they are different in concept from mercury zinc cells. The first Greatbatch cell was a solid state type. It didn't have liquid electrolytes. It looked bulky, and big as compared with other cells, however, it marked the beginning of a new era in pacemaker energy: the lithium power. Well, as of now, there is a variety of lithium cells available (Figure

TYPE	MANUFACTURER	CAPACITY
IODINE	WG, CRC	1.5-4 Ah @ 2.8 V
SILVER CHROMATE	SAFT	0.5 Ah @ 3.45V
THIONYL CHLORIDE	GTE	2.0 Ah @ 3.6 V
LEAD IODIDE	MALLORY	0.9 Ah @ 5.7 V
BROMINE	WG (Development)	3.5 Ah @ 3.45V

Figure 8. Types and energy capacities of various lithium cells.

8). There is Mallory, the General Telephone Electric Company, Catalyst Research Corporation, and well, one more is the Saft cell. Figure 9 shows a cutaway of the Greatbatch 702E lithium iodide cell just to give you an idea of what is inside. There is a metallic lithium anode inside the sandwich-like con-

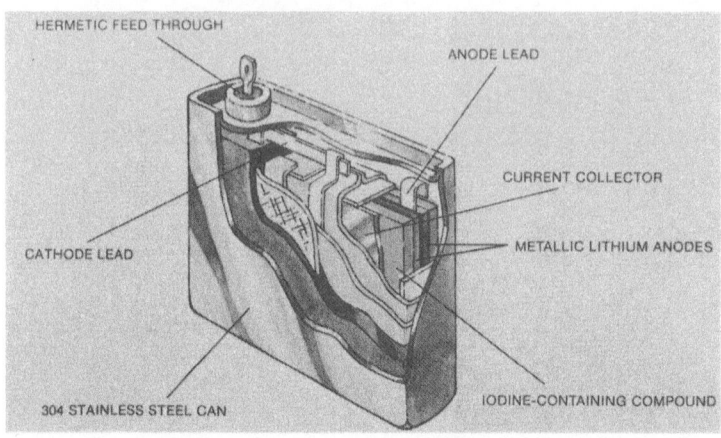

Figure 9. Cutaway view of 702E lithium cell (courtesy CPI).

struction and the two outside cathodes are made of iodine. In between there is polyvinyl pyridine compounded with lithium iodide as an electrolyte to serve as a medium for ionic conduction. The two metal-like substances are spaced with a non-corrosive lithium iodine compound. It's crystalline and the electricity flows in ionic form to the metal anode. There is no gas evolving as a by-product of this reaction nor metal particles penetrating the separator because the separator and electrolyte are solid state. The only byproduct is lithium iodide and that appears in increased amount as the battery is depleted. Almost all lithium anode mass converts into lithium iodide with cell depletion. This battery can be hermetically sealed as opposed to mercury zinc batteries which cannot because during the process of discharge they evolve hydrogen gas. This is an additional advantage, and has made lithium cells more and more popular. The chemical reaction of the lithium cell is $2Li + I_2 = 2LiI + e$. We have lithium metal converting to lithium ions and electrons and these lithium ions combine with iodine to form lithium iodide, the same material which is serving as solid electrolyte. Thus, there are no volatile discharge byproducts nor corrosive reactants within the cell, hence its greater reliability and lack of catastrophic failure modes.

The Saft cell (Figure 10) has a different construction than the Wilson Greatbatch cell and is a later cell on the market. It was introduced in 1973 for medical use but has been in military and watch use in France and all over Europe since 1970. The Saft cell is a lithium-silver chromate cell and contains a lithium metallic anode. Lithium perchlorate serves as electrolyte dissolved in propylene carbonate, and the cathode is made of silver chromate, powder and graphite. This cell, similar to the Wilson Greatbatch cell does not have a catastrophic failure mechanism. There is no possibility of internal shorts or corrosion. There

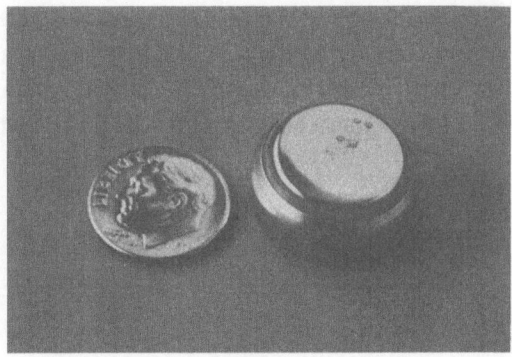

Figure 10. Photograph of Saft lithium cell (courtesy CPI).

are no corrosive materials unless there is some impurity, especially water which may get in during the manufacturing process. Lithium is very highly reactive with water, so these cells require very stringent quality control measures to prevent water and other impurities from getting inside the cell. A crossection of

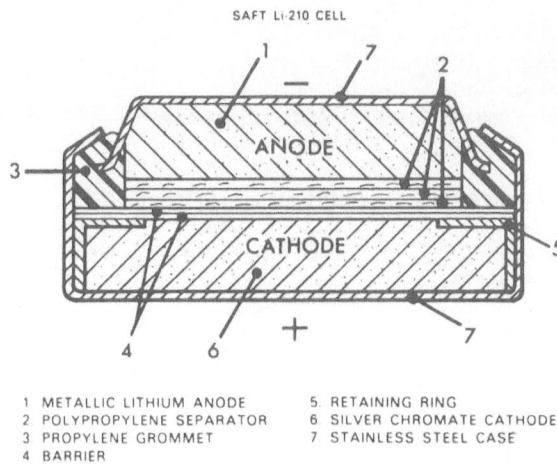

SAFT Li-210 CELL

1 METALLIC LITHIUM ANODE   5. RETAINING RING
2 POLYPROPYLENE SEPARATOR   6. SILVER CHROMATE CATHODE
3 PROPYLENE GROMMET   7. STAINLESS STEEL CASE
4 BARRIER

Figure 11. Cross section of Saft cell (courtesy CPI).

the Saft lithium cell (Figure 11) shows the lithium anode and silver chromate cathode and this is the pacemaker cell used in the Saft pacemaker powered devices. It has a pellet construction with a separator in between the anode and cathode. The performance characteristic of the Wilson Greatbatch 702E cell, as compared with the Saft cell is depicted on Figure 12 and 13. Ideally we would like to have a cell which would provide straight line performance over a period of time and then would gradually drop down when depleted. This is not the case. Some of the energy cannot be drawn from the cell, and under micro ampere loads, there is a slow decline of voltage common to all chemical cells. A certain amount of energy is wasted inside of the cell for internal leakage or for charge transfer and other electro-chemical mechanisms. All cells exhibit a drop off in the

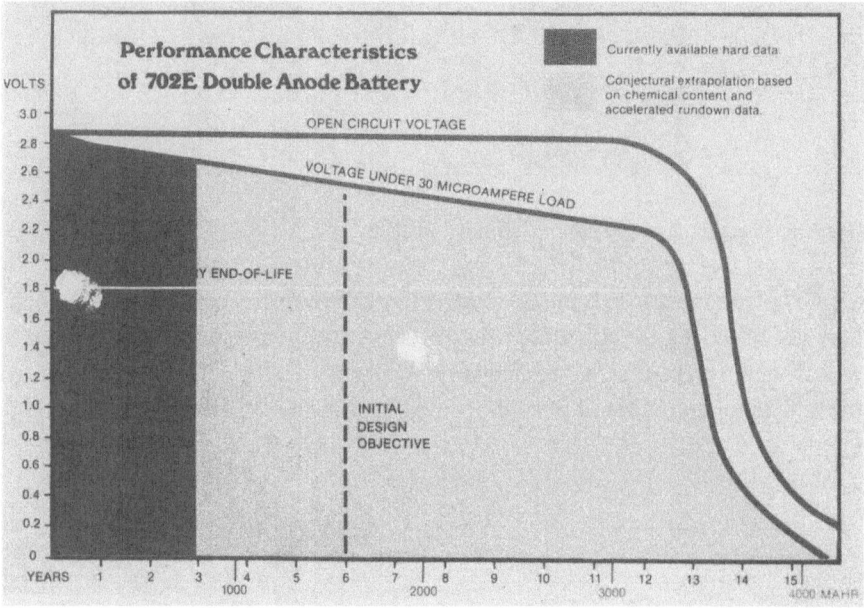

Figure 12. Discharge curve of 702E Greatbatch lithium cell (courtesy CPI).

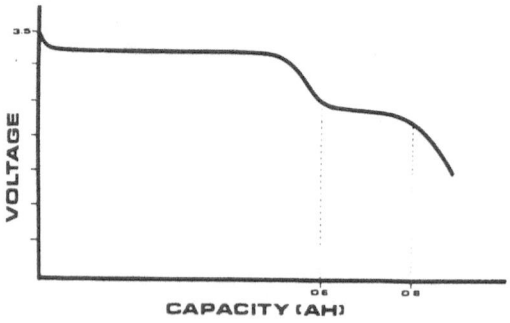

Figure 13. Discharge curve of Saft lithium cell (courtesy CPI).

voltage delivered vs. time. A comparison of the performance of lithium and mercury cells is shows on Figure 14. This figure gives an idea of how to compare the various cells. If there was no cell discharge and no waste mechanism in the cell, the line would be parallel to the bottom line and straight. Lithium has much lower internal waste or internal leakage than mercury. That is why the slope of usable energy is less steep than that for mercury cell. The internal discharge mechanism of the cell is responsible for many of them failing earlier than predicted (or rated capacity). If the given current drain is known, one can draw a line representing the current drain vs. time. The battery would be depleted when these

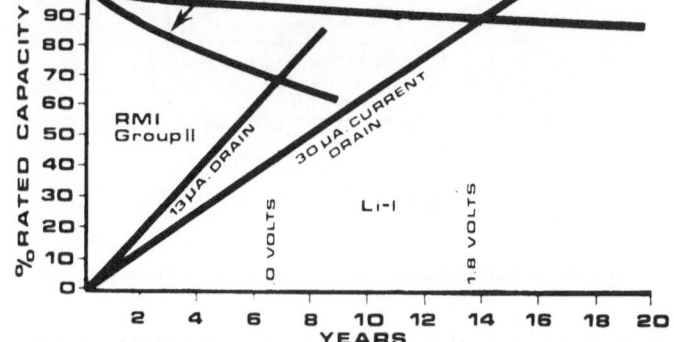

Figure 14. Performance characteristics of lithium iodide vs. improved mercury zinc cell (courtesy CPI).

two lines intersect. That would represent total depletion and the battery voltage would drop down to 0 volts. This graph is optimistic for Group II mercury cells, but it shows how to go about comparing the internal losses in the cell vs. current drain. For lithium powered pacemakers, the current drain from the cell is generally higher. One of the reasons for the higher current drain from the circuit is that the batteries do not deliver high enough voltage for pacing, so their voltage has to be doubled by electronic means. This is because the lithium cells are big and inconvenient to put in series in most cases, while mercury batteries have been used in series, and you can stack them up to get a desired voltage. On Figure 14 we can compare an approximation of generator life showing the conventional mercury zinc battery powered pacemaker's longevity somewhere in the order of two to three years, lithium lasting much longer up to six to seven years or longer depending upon the cell type.

Nuclear energy sources

There are two basic types of nuclear cells. The Beta cell is a nuclear cell which contains radioactive promethium where beta radiation energy is converted directly into electricity. The plutonium cell is a nuclear cell containing a radioactive plutonium compound. In Figure 15 we see a cross section of a nuclear powered

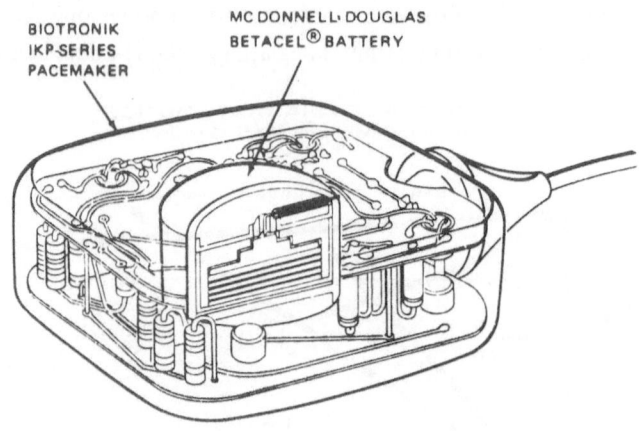

Figure 15. Cutaway view of Betacel pacemaker powered by promethium (Biotronik).

pacemaker using the promethium or Beta cell made by McDonald Douglas. This pacemaker is on its way out. Its longevity is in the order of five to eight years and thus offers rather little advantage over lithium pacemakers with all of the disadvantages of nuclear pacemakers in terms of tracing, radiation, protection, regulations, administrative problems, licensing problems, and so on.

Another energy source which is still growing in use is a plutonium cell. Radioactive decay of plutonium generates heat which heats the thermopile to generate electricity. This is an indirect energy conversion from nuclear decay to heat and to electricity. The advantage of this source is its longevity. The half life of plutonium is close to 87 years and as such, the plutonium capsule can generate energy for the lifetime of the patient. The complexity of shielding the radiation and shielding the heat and converting it into electricity has been successfully resolved by manufacturers, and this pacemaker is the most highly reliable product ever made by man today. They have been tested to the greatest possible hazards of cremation, impact, crashes, and vibrations for reliability and have passed these tests required by the Nuclear Regulatory Commission for Public Safety. The only disadvantage is the expense and the very complex technology and book keeping necessary to implement the application. Figure 16 is an example of a plutonium pacemaker made by Coratomic, a United States firm, which is to my knowledge the most handsome and smallest pacemaker on the market using a nuclear cell.

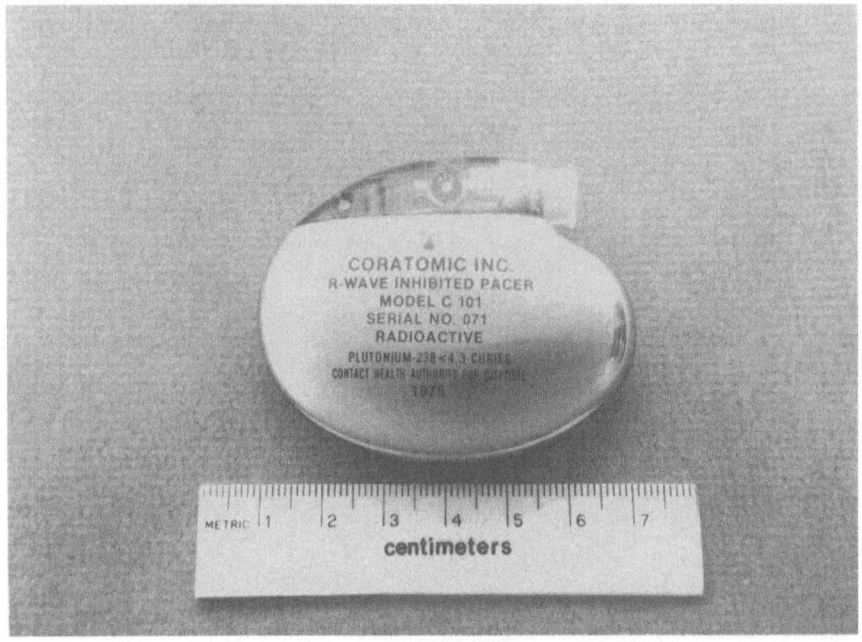

Figure 16. External appearance of nuclear pacemaker powered by plutonium (courtesy Noah Sexton Coratomic).

Future trends

There is another group of devices using different energy sources including biogalvanic which have not been used yet clinically on a great scale, although have been tried clinically. Figure 17 shows the biogalvanic pacemaker, which I've been involved in. During my engineering career, I have devoted at least half of my productive years to the development of biogalvanic pacemakers. I am show-ing you for your interest what other energy choice the future may bring. This is a pacemaker which, theoretically, also can serve for a patient's lifetime. It has platinum black outside covers which are biocompatible and do not cause the tissue reaction phenomena earlier experienced by Dr. Schaldach in his clinical trials on his biogalvanic pacers. Our pacemakers have been implanted in dogs for over two and a half years and are performing as expected. They do exhibit a very slow voltage decay curve as all batteries do. The problem is to determine where this decay curve drops below an acceptable level. This pacemaker cell is physi-cally an open system and is not a hermetically sealed battery. Only the circuitry is hermetically sealed. The biogalvanic cell produces a low voltage while using oxygen ions from the interstitial tissue fluid to generate electrical power. Thus, it has virtually an unlimited source of energy. The only limitation is the buildup of the tissue reaction, which I believe we have overcome and also the buildup of

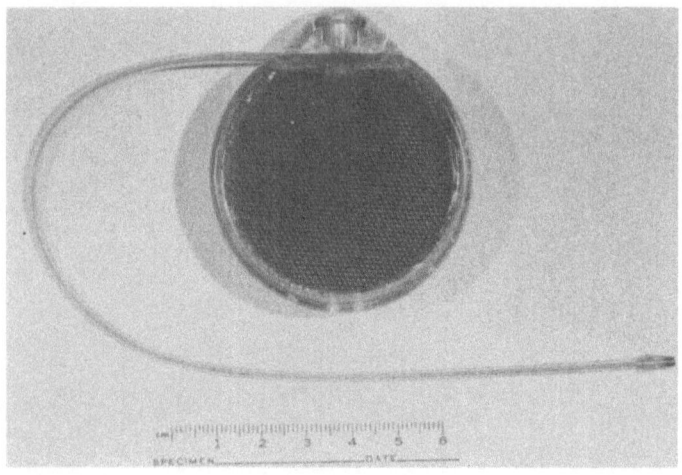

Figure 17. External appearance of a biogalvanic pacemaker (Cywinski).

protein layers deactivating the platinum catalyst surface. This latter factor is probably responsible for cell voltage decay which is nevertheless very slow (ca 10 mv/year.

In conclusion, I would like to emphasize that my remarks have concentrated in the factors reflecting on longevity of the pacemaker as determined by the energy source. As new cells appear on the market, both improved mercury zinc cells, lithium cells, and nuclear cells, the reliability and total longevity of the pacemaker system may no longer solely depend on the longevity of the power source. The power source may become one of the more reliable components in the pacemaker system. From an engineering point of view, I would like to mention some figures giving a comparison done by the military industry on the reliability of some of the electronic components which are included in pacemaker generators. In probable number of failure on a scale of $\times 10^{-9}$ per hour, the ceramic capacitor, which is a very common component in the pacemaker circuit, has a 100 rating. The resistor is the most reliable component, and it has a 20 rating and thus has a probability of 20×10^{-9} failures per hour. The transistor has a 6,000 rating and the tantalum capacitor which is commonly used as the output capacitor in pacemakers has a 2,000 rating. As compared to those ratings, the Saft lithium cell has a rating of 80 and the Mallory mercury cell has a rating of 2,000.

So you can see the range of expected reliability and random failures during the predicted lifetime of the power source and the pacemaker circuit. What is the ideal power source for a pacemaker? I would put in first place high reliability and in this instance it seems that both nuclear and lithium have an edge over others. The maximum energy capacity or density per volume and per weight is important. Well, again in that aspect, lithium seems to lead the way. The battery should be capable of being hermetically sealed. Again, lithium and nuclear batteries are capable of this. The battery should exhibit minimum internal losses. Time will tell how well lithium will score in this regard. They should provide high voltage or high electromotive force, open circuit. None of the batteries, except for a few experimental ones has yet matched the five volt output directly from the cell. The battery should exhibit a reliable depletion indication for eventual replacement. The lithium silver chromate cell has the best indicator to my knowledge of impending depletion. It has a two voltage level; when it is 80 percent depleted, it switches to lower voltage output, and it has still 20 percent capacity left.

Well, this concludes my presentation, and I would like to say that other long life batteries are still under development and investigation and if the price can be reasonable, they may appear on the market. I would like to close quoting J. Galsworthy, 'Those who do not think about the future do not have one,' and that is what we engineers have been doing all along.

Literature

Auborn, J. and Marincic, N., Inorganic Electrolyte Lithium Cells. *Power Sources 5* Academic Press, New York 683-694, 1975.

Cataldi, H., Performance of a Mercuric Oxide-Zinc Battery Specifically Designed for Implantable Cardiac Pulse Generators. *10th AAMI Meeting.* Boston, MA. 1975.

Hahn, A., Cooper, J., Cywinski, J., Salkind, A., Implanted Hybrid Cells for Biological Power Applications. *Proc. Electrochemical Society Conference.* Atlantic City, N.J., 203-205, 1970.

Cywinski, J., Hahn, A., Cooper, J., Implantable Transmitters Powered by Bio-Galvanic Cells. *Proc. 1972 San Diego Biomedical Symposium.* 113-120, 1972.

Cywinski, J., Cooper, J., Hahn, A., Biogalvanic Power Sources. *Proceedings IVth International Symposium on Cardiac Pacing, Groningen 1973.* Royal Van Gorcum, Assen 216-220, 1974.

Cywinski, J., Advances in Cardiac Pacemakers – New Power Sources and Circuit Technology, *IEEE Intercon 75.* New York 1975.

Cywinski, J., Currently Available Energy Sources for Cardiac Pacemakers: A Review, *Proceedings of the Pacemaker Colloquium,* Norman J. and Rickards, A., Eds. Vitatron Medical, Arnhem 87, 1976.

Cywinski, J., Hahn, A., Easley, J., Performance of Implanted Biogalvanic Pacemakers, *Proceedings Vth International Symposium on Cardiac Pacing.* Tokyo 1976, Excerpta Medica, Amsterdam 447-451, 1977.

Doty, R., Fester, K., Long Term Experience with Improved Power Sources for Implantable Devices. *Proc. Ann. Conf. Eng. Med. Biol.* Bal Harbour, Florida 308, 1972.

Fester, K., Doty, R., Velden, R., Symposium on Energy Alternatives. *Proc. 16th Ann. American Soc. Mechanical Engineers,* New Mexico 1976.

Fester, K., Doty, R., Effects of Epoxy Encapsulation on Performance of Pacemaker Batteries. *8th*

Ann. AAMI Meeting, Washington D.C. 1973.

Gasper, K., Fester, K., Cardiac Pacemaker Power Sources. *Proc. Intersociety Energy Conversion Engineering Conf.* Newark, Del. 1205-1213, 1975.

Lehmann, G., Rassinoux, T., Gerbier, G., Gabano, J., The Silver Chromate-Lithium Cell. *Power Sources 4.* Oriel Press, 299-307, 1973.

Love, J., Lewis, K., Fischell, R., The Johns Hopkins Rechargeable Pacemaker. *JAMA,*234-1, 64-66, 1975.

Marincic, N., Epstein, J., Goebel, F., Lombardi, A., Lithium Inorganic Battery for Cardiac Pacemaker Application. *Extended Abstracts.* 75, 2, Electrochem. Soc., Dallas, Texas 101-102, 1973.

Ruben, S., Sealed Zinc-Mercuric Oxide Cells for Implantable Cardiac Pacemakers. *Ann. New York Acad. Sci.* 627-634, 1969.

CORONARY SINUS PACING
INDICATIONS AND CLINICAL PROBLEMS

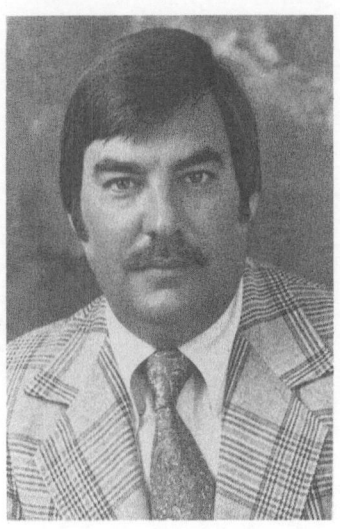

Dr. John Messenger received his undergraduate education at the University of Dayton in 1959 and his medical degree at the University of Cincinnati School of Medicine in 1963. Following internship at Los Angeles County Harbor General Hospital and two years of medical residency at Wadsworth General V.A. Hospital, he spent two further years of cardiac fellowship at the University of California in Los Angeles. He became Director of the Coronary Care Unit of the Wadsworth General V.A. Hospital in 1971 and Acting Chief of Cardiology in 1972. Since 1973 he has been Director of Critical Care Medicine at Memorial Hospital Medical Center, Long Beach, California. He has an active interest in the management of cardiac arrhythmias in the acute and chronic situation and has published several papers in related areas.

CORONARY SINUS PACING
INDICATIONS AND CLINICAL PROBLEMS

JOHN D. MESSENGER, M.D. AND MYRVIN H. ELLESTAD, M.D.

In 1970, Moss et al. reported on 14 patients with a variety of arrhythmias, including supraventricular tachycardia and bradycardia-tachycardia syndrome, using special bipolar leads in the coronary sinus as a reliable method of atrial pacing (1). This study concluded that the coronary sinus is a reliable method of atrial pacing without resorting to thoracotomy.

The physiology of the atrial contribution to the cardiac output has been well documented (2, 8). A recent publication by Guyton demonstrates a significant reduction in cardiac output (22%), with loss of the atrial mechanism following open heart surgery in patient with impaired ventricular function (right ventriculotomy) when compared with a control group of post cardiac surgery patients (without ventriculotomy). Cardiac output decreases 5% (p less than 0.01)

Selection of patients

1. In our patient population 20-25% of potential electrophysiologic problems appear to be candidates for some variety of atrial pacing.

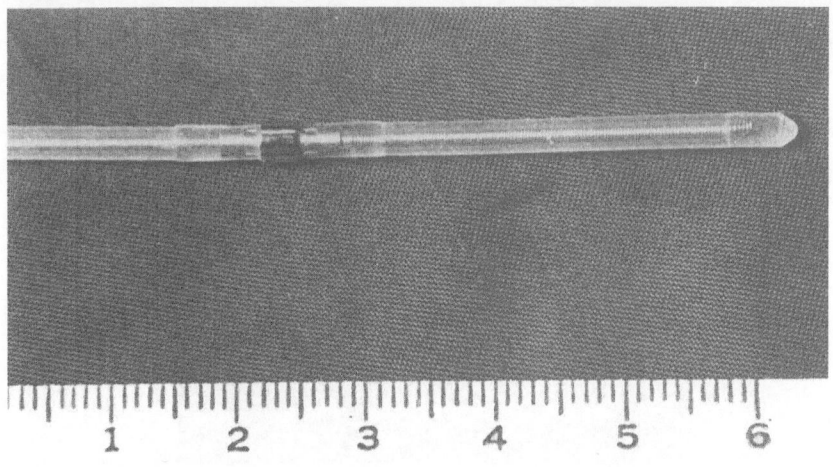

Figure 1. Cordis Coronary Sinus Unipolar Electrode.

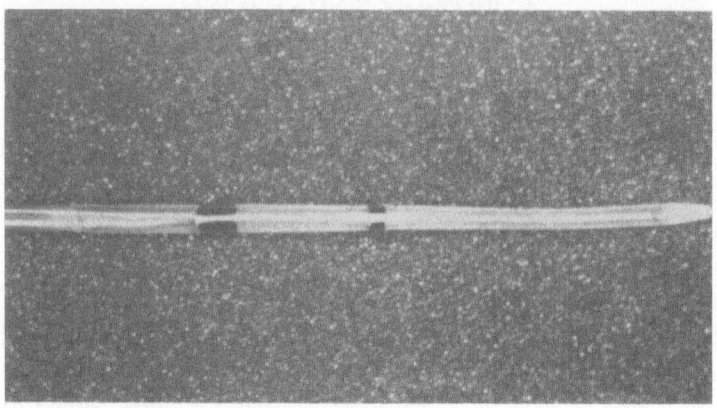

Figure 2. Medtronic Bipolar Coronary Sinus Electrode.
             (Special lead – not commercially available)

2. Atrial pacing study and his bundle recording are prerequisites to placement of
    permanent atrial leads.

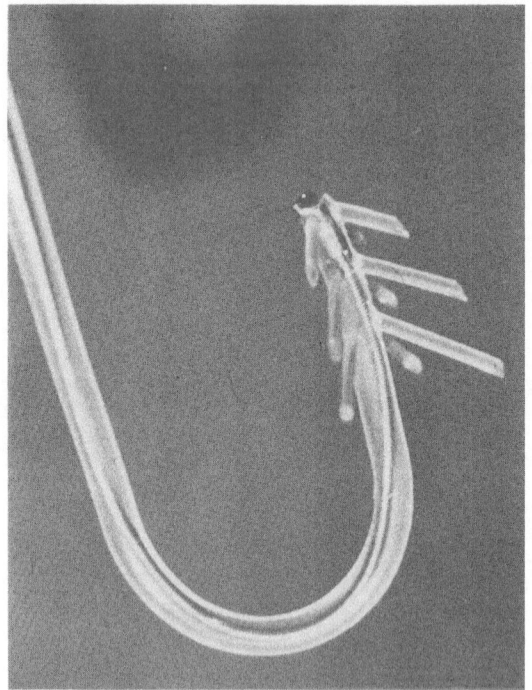

Figure 3. Medtronic Unipolar 'tined' J lead for positioning in atrial appendage.

During the past 8 years, the search for a reliable atrial electrode has spawned a number of developments and techniques to achieve various therapeutic goals where atrial pacing is preferred to ventricular pacing (10, 14). A variety of lead systems for atrial stimulation have been introduced and include the unipolar lead with a 'tail' produced by Cordis (Fig. 1) and a bipolar electrode with a 'tail' specially made by Medtronic (Fig. 2). Each of these leads is intended for positioning in the coronary sinus. Other leads intended for positioning in the atrial appendage include spring anchor leads, 'J' electrodes, and the tined 'J' lead of Medtronic (Fig. 3).

The purpose of this paper is to describe the indications and problems of permanent coronary sinus pacing in a broad spectrum of patients presenting to our hospital with the clinical conditions indicated in Table 1.

Table 1

A.   *Sinus Node Dysfunction* (Intact AV Conduction System)
  1.   Periodic sinus bradycardia due to SA arrest; existing block with periods of asystole with normal sinus recovery time (SRT).
  2.   Sick sinus syndrome: Sinus bradycardia with prolonged SRT.
  3.   Bradycardia-tachycardia syndrome: in combination with suppressive drugs.
  4.   Chronotropic incompetence (CI): inappropriate rate response (autonomic mediation)
     a.   Coronary artery disease; anginal syndrome when Inderal cannot be used due to extremely slow rate.
     b.   Valvular disease: aortic insufficiency and mitral insufficiency (nonsurgical candidates). By increasing the rate, the hemodynamic status can frequently be improved.
     c.   Congestive heart failure: increased cardiac output in raterelated endstage myocardial failure.
  5.   Recurrent supraventricular tachycardia.
B.   *Recurrent Ventricular Tachycardia*
C.   *Complete Heart Block with Low Output Syndrome*

Method

The technique of placement of a coronary sinus electrode has been described in prior publications (1, 12). Both right and left cephalic and right and left external jugular approaches were used. The catheters were Cordis unipolar coronary sinus catheters or Medtronic bipolar coronary sinus catheters (Table 2).

Competency of AV conduction was ascertained utilizing transvenous pacer in the coronary sinus or in the atrium along with intracavitary recordings, atrial pacing studies, sinus recovery times and HIS bundle recordings when indicated. Fluroscopic positioning was used in all cases along with simultaneous surface

Table 2

1.	Variability in anatomy of coronary sinus may pose technical problems.
2.	Threshold – Less than 3 m.a. acceptable
3.	Sensing – proximal location gives greatest sensing
	A. P-waves usually less than 2 mv
	B. R-wave usually displays low voltage thus high sensitivity sensing circuits are required.
	C. Lack of fixation causes variable pacing and sensing (trombone slide effect) and loss of tissue-electrode contact. Potentially, this could induce atrial and/or ventricular arrhythmias.
	D. PR interval not to exceed 0.24-0.26 seconds, ideally less than 0.20

electrogram plus coronary vein electrogram. Thresholds were measured in proximal, middle and distal coronary sinus. During the past two years, recordings and thresholds have been made with Medtronic and/or Cordis Pacer Systems Analyzer.

Indications and results   (Table 3)

Sixty-eight patients have been followed who have had permanent pervenous coronary sinus pacing with a range of two months to six years (average 21.4 months). The greatest majority of these patients have been implanted since the introduction of the Cordis Rate Adjustable (RA) Pacer, and a significant number of Medtronic (RA) pacers have been utilized during the time as part of the clinical validation.

Table 3

1.	Bradycardia	25 Patients
2.	Bradycardia-Tachycardia Syndrome	26 Patients
3.	Low Cardiac Output and Bradycardia (Chronotropic Incompetence)	10 Patients
4.	Supraventricular Tachycardia 'Orthorhythmic Mode'	2 Patients
5.	Recurrent Ventricular Tachycardia	4 Patients
6.	Complete Heart Block (Coronary Sinus Lead) with Low Output Syndrome	1 Patient
		68 Patients

Bradycardia, which includes patients with persistent bradycardia, intermittent SA arrest, and SA block with documented associated symptoms of syncope or transient ischemic attacks. This group of twenty-five patients consists of those with both normal and abnormal sinus recovery time.

Bradycardia-tachycardia syndrome. Twenty-six patients were implanted with excellent clinical results. A prior history of multiple admissions to the hospital for symptomatic tachycardia, 'refractory' to standard therapy was required prior to implantation of an atrial electrode.

Of the fifty-one patients in these two classifications, only two of these patients required a change of electrode; one to the ventricle and one had a right atrial 'pinch-on' electrode placed via thoracotomy. Both of these problems resulted from excessive and unexplained rise in stimulation threshold.

Low output syndrome and bradycardia were noted in 10 patients with a variety of disorders, i.e., aortic incompetence, mitral insufficiency, cardiomyopathy, and ischemic myocardial dysfunction. The majority of these patients underwent cardiac catherization and hemodynamic data confirmed significant reduction in cardiac output. All had inappropriate rate response which we have termed chronotropic incompetence (CI). The addition of atrial 'kick' and rate increase with RA pacers, has lead to improvement of at least one clinical cardiac classification of the American Heart Association. One patient in this group (cardiomyopathy) progressed to complete heart block two years after implant necessitating a revision to a right ventricular electrode. One patient recently died 28 months after implant of progressive neurological disease. The myocardium was not implicated. (No post mortem).

Supraventricular tachycardia (SVT). Two patients with recurrent SVT have had implants. With the pacer in magnet mode, asynchronous pacing has repeatedly interrupted these recurrent tachycardias. A special design pacer (Cordis) was made for the second patient with a repetition rate of 220 BPM in magnet mode. Both patients continue to do well clinically. The addition of the coronary sinus pacer has permitted greater dosages of beta blockers to be used in both patients, but SVT has continued to occur intermittently.

Recurrent ventricular tachycardia. There are four patients in this group, all of whom have had angiographic and hemodynamic studies. Two patients were operated with coronary artery bypass grafts and aneurysmectomy with persistent ventricular tachycardia; one followed acute MI and the fourth was a cardiomyopathy. One of these patients has been explanted (the only explant in the series), and one was converted to a right ventricular position due to increase in threshold. All of these have required a regimen of multiple antiarrhythmias in addition to pacing.

Complete heart block with low output syndrome (with sinus rhythm). Only one patient has had coronary sinus and right ventricular leads as the initial implant, utilizing a Cordis Omni Atricor pacemaker. This patient has done extremely well clinically.

Complications and problems (Major) (see Table 4)

Table 4

1.	Deaths – 3 all late, more than 12 months after implant
	1 Acute MI documented, more than one year after implant. Coronary sinus pacer continued to function. (No post mortem)
	1 Progressive neurological symptoms, Parkinsonism and pneumonia. Pacer noted to function in IMCU. (No post mortem)
	1 Unknown cause. (No post mortem)
2.	Coronary Sinus Perforation and/or Obstruction
	0 This remains a theoretical complication.
3.	Dislodgement – Total (Standard RV Lead)
	1 Requiring placement in right ventricle
4.	Repositioning required – in coronary sinus
	4 During initial hospitalization with good long terms results
5.	Relocation due to development of excessively high thresholds – 3
	1 Placed epicardially right atrium
	2 Right ventricle
6.	Relocation to right ventricle due to development of complete heart block
	1 Two years after initial implant

Minor

7.	Intermittent sensing noted not requiring repositioning or revision. No clinical significance to date other than variable rate.
	7
8.	Recurrent episodes of supraventricular tachycardias requiring hospitalization; 2 required DC cardioversion
	4
9.	Digitalis toxicity manifested by prolongation of PR interval and high serum digoxin level; returned toward normal after digoxin discontinued.
	2

1. *Deaths*: 3/68 deaths have occurred, all late, more than 12 months after initial implant. One patient suffered an acute myocardial infarction, and the coronary sinus pacer continued to function. However, the terminal event was ventricular tachycardia-ventricular fibrillation. The second patient succumbed of a stroke four years after the coronary sinus pacer implantation, and the third succumbed of pneumonia and advanced Parkinson's Disease. Unfortunately, no post mortem was obtained in any of these cases. The status of the coronary sinus electrode in vivo remains unknown to us.

2. Coronary sinus perforation and/or obstruction has not occurred to date in any of our patients; however, it remains a theoretical complication. The use of special electrodes with tapered, softened tips most likely increases the safety of this procedure.

3. *Dislodgement*. One of 68 dislodged and required placement in the right ven-

tricle. This was an 'early' implant and utilized a standard right ventricular electrode.

4. Repositioning in the coronary sinus was required in 4/68 (16%). This was heralded by loss of capture, and/or loss of sensing, causing significant competition and/or reduction in rate. All occurred within the first few days post implant, and all were successfully repositioned.

5. Relocation of the electrode, due to development of excessively high threshold, occurred in 3/68 (4%) necessitating two to be placed in the right ventricle and the third to be placed by thoracotomy with an atrial 'pinch on' lead. Investigation of the coronary sinus during repositioning revealed a threshold increase of greater than 9 m.a. in all position. The reason for this remains unknown.

6. Relocation to the right ventricle, due to development of complete heart block, occurred in one patient two years after implant. This is the only instance 1/68 (1.5%) of complete heart block in our series. Bundle branch block with intact AV nodal function has appeared in several patients.

Complications and problems (Minor)

7. Intermittent sensing noted in 7/68 (10%). This has occurred presumably by three mechanisms:
    A. R-wave voltage was inadequate for the sensing circuit, and competition has occurred. The theoretical development of tachyarrhythmia remains a possibility, as four patients have had recurrent tachyarrhythmia. The problem has been overcome by utilizing Cordis 'high' sensitivity RA pacer, when R-waves measure less than 4 mv.
    B. The short refractory period of the standard pacemaker circuit has caused changing rates and irregular rhythms, due to sensing of the following QRs in patients with prolonged P-R intervals.
    C. Occasionally, we have observed significant motion of the coronary sinus electrode, sliding in and out of the coronary sinus, which may contribute to these abnormalities. None of the electrodes have been repositioned or removed.

8. Recurrent episodes of SVT/atrial fibrillation, requiring hospitalization. 4/26 (15%) of the tachy-brady group, have required hospitalization: two necessitated cardioversion and two spontaneously converted. Loss of sensing was noted in one patient during atrial fibrillation, which reverted following cardioversion.

9. Digitalis toxicity has occurred in 2/64 (3%) of the patients. Prolongation of the PR interval and Wenchebach occurred in one case, associated with abnormally high serum Digoxin levels. Both cases reverted towards normal PR interval following discontinuance of Digoxin.

Observations and conclusions

1. Over a six year period, sixty-eight patients have had coronary sinus permanent electrodes and generators. The majority of implants have occurred following the development of rate adjustable (RA) Cordis pacemakers (1972). Successful implants: 62/68 (93%) for long term pacing. Four required relocation of the electrode to another site, and one was explanted. Thus, the coronary sinus provides a safe, stable location for long term atrial pacing.

2. As has been shown previously, (Moss et al.) (1, 12), chronic rise in thresholds is usually less than 1.5 m.a. (confirmed by our experience).

3. Antiarrhythmic agents have been used in combination with coronary sinus pacing with a significant reduction in readmission for recurrent tachycardias (only 4/24) in our group to date (17%).

4. Utilization of coronary sinus/atrial pacing in patients with low output syndrome (CHF), associated with bradycardia, has markedly improved this group clinically by at least one functional American Heart Association classification confirming the importance of atrial contribution and rate contribution in individuals with significant ventricular dysfunction.

5. New designs in pacemaker electronics are required to enhance atrial/coronary sinus pacing techniques. Special generators with improved *sensing* circuits (less than 1 mv), and longer refractory periods (more than 400 milliseconds), are required. Redesign of coronary sinus electrodes to provide more surface interface may be of help and experimental models are now being developed.

Literature

1. Kramer, D.H., Moss, A.J., Permanent pervenous atrial pacing from the coronary vein. *Circulation* 42, 427-436, 1970.
2. Brockman, S.K., Dynamic function of atrial contraction in regulation of cardiac performance. *Am. J. Physiol.* 203, 597, 1963.
3. Parker, J.O., Ledwich J.R., West, R.O., Case R.B., Reversible cardiac failure during angina pectoris. Hemodynamic effects of atrial pacing in coronary artery disease. *Circulation* 39, 745, 1969.

4. Brockman, S.K. et al, Physiologic studies and clinical experience in patients with synchronous and asynchronous pacemakers. *J. Thoracic and Cardiovascular Surg.* 51, 864, 1965.
   Martin, R.H. and Cobb, L.H., Observation on the effect of atrial systole in men. *J. Lab. Clin. Med.* 68, 224, 1966.

6. Wisehart, J. D., Wright, J.E.C., Rosenfeldt, F.L. and Ross, J.H., Atrial and ventricular pacing after open heart surgery. *Thorax* 28, 9-14, 1973.

7. Benchimol, A., Ellis, J.G., Dimond, E.G., Hemodynamic consequences of atrial and ventricular pacing in patients with normal and abnormal hearts. Effect of exercise at a fixed atrial and ventricular rate. *Am. J. Med.* 39, 911, 1965.

8. Karlof, I., Haemodynamic effect of atrial triggered versus fixed rate pacing at rest and during exercise in complete heart block. *acta Med. Scand.* 197, 195-206, 1975.

9. Guyton, R.A., Andrews, J.M., Hickey, P.R., Michaelis, L.L., Morris, A.G., The contribution of atrial contraction to right heart function before and after right ventriculotomy. *J. Thoracic and Cardiovascular Surg.* 71, 1-10, 1976.

10. Furman, S., Therapeutic uses of atrial pacing. *Am. Heart J.* 6, 835-840, 1973.

11. Dreifus, L.S., Berkovitz, B.V., Kimibiris, D., Moghadam, K., Haupt, G., Walinsky, P., Thomas, P., Brockman, S.K., Use of atrial and bifocal cardiac pacemakers for treating resistant dysrhythmias. *Eur. J. Cardiol.* 3, 257-266, 1975.

12. Moss, A.J., Therapeutic uses of permanent pervenous atrial pacemakers: A Review. *J. Electrocardiology* 8, 373-380, 1975.

13. Lajos, T.Z., Wanka, J., Transvenous atrial pacing with a new electrode. *J. Thoracic and Cardiovascular Surg.* 69, 575-578, 1975.

14. Moore, C.B., Bower, P.B., The sick sinus syndrome. *S. Med. J.* 68, 32-78, 1975.

TEMPORARY PACING: METHODS AND COMPLICATIONS

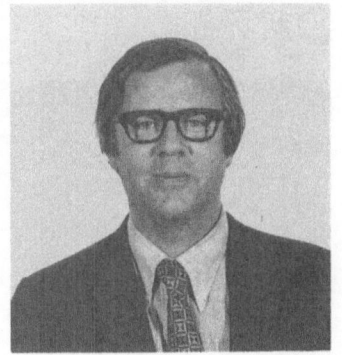

Dr. Thomas A. Preston is presently Associate Professor of Medicine at the University of Washington, Seattle Washington and Co-Director of Cardiology at the U.S. Public Health Service Hospital in Seattle. His dual background with a degree in electrical engineering as well as in medicine has made him particularly well adapted to lecture and write on various aspects of cardiac pacing. He is the recipient of many awards which attest to his ability as a teacher. He is a Fellow of the American College of Cardiology and the American Heart Association Council on Clinical Cardiology. He is the author of several papers dealing with electrical stimulation of the heart and a recent book on coronary artery surgery.

TEMPORARY PACING: METHODS AND COMPLICATIONS

THOMAS PRESTON, M.D.

Indications

The major indications for temporary pacing are illustrated in Figure 1, including both ventricular and atrial pacing. If feasible and reliable, atrial pacing is often the preferable mode. Ventricular bradycardia or asystole due either to complete heart block or cardiac standstill constituted the major indication for pacing ten to fifteen years ago. The general experience is that these indications have decreased relative to other indications and probably less than a quarter of all temporary pacers are now inserted for either complete heart block or asystole. We employ temporary pacing much more with other clinical situations, as the usage of pacemakers becomes better delineated. Bradycardia of any sort, e.g. sinus node block, sinus bradycardia or arrest with a slow escape rhythm, is an indication for temporary pacing if it is causing a hemodynamic problem or syncope.

INDICATIONS FOR TEMPORARY PACING

I. Bradycardia
  1. Complete heart block
  2. Second degree, or high-grade A-V block
  3. S.-A- bradycardia, block, or arrest
  4. Impending bradycardia (acute myocardial infarction, anesthesia)
II. Tachycardia
  1. Supra-ventricular
    a. Paroxysmal SVT (atrial or junctional)
    b. Non-paroxysmal SVT
    c. Artial flutter
  2. Ventricular tachycardia
III. Diagnostic tests
  1. Stress test for angina
  2. Electrophysiologic pacing studies
IV. Other
  1. Post-op (open heart) low output syndrome
  2. Protection during coronary arteriography

We have already heard something about the use of pacing with tachycardias. There are two basic physiologic mechanisms of pacing for tachycardias. One is called overdrive pacing, which Dr. Zoll alluded to in which the pacing rate is faster than the underlying sinus, junctional or ventricular rate. If used to suppress ectopic beats, the overdriving pacing interval need not necessarily be shorter than the interval between the sinus beat and the premature ectopic ventricular beat. Overdrive pacing simply means capturing the heart through pacing and driving it at a rate somewhat above the basic underlying natural rate. Interruption pacing is used in treatment of re-entry type arrhythmias, wherein a single properly timed pacing stimulus, or perhaps two or three stimuli can interrupt the re-entry type arrhythmia and convert it to sinus rhythm. These pacing techniques are applicable to sustained tachycardias or to ectopic activity with premature beats occurring in salvos. Pacing to control tachycardias is most commonly used in Coronary Care Units.

Ventricular irritability especially may occur as a result of drugs. The phenothiazines and tricyclicamines may cause ventricular irritability. Drug therapy of drug induced arrhythmias is often unsuccessful and in such cases pacing, either atrial or ventricular, may be remarkably successful. The prolonged Q-T syndrome is another example in which pacing can be very successful, either for short term or long term therapy.

We must consider pre-heart block syndromes which arise in two special situations: acute myocardial infarction and anesthesia. Let me dispense with the second one first. Five or more years ago there was great interest in the situation in which the patient facing general anesthesia had the combination of right bundle branch block and left axis deviation (bifascicular block). It was unknown whether these patients should have prophylactic temporary pacing during anesthesia. The general experience is that this has been unnecessary, and there have been several clinical studies supporting this position. Unless there are other indications of prior second or third degree block, or indications that the patient has been symptomatic due to bradyarrhythmias, in general, these pre-heart block syndromes do not require the use of temporary pacing during anesthesia. If there is a reasonable question prior to surgery, one might do an electro-physiologic study, although this requires more effort and time than placing a prophylactic temporary catheter.

There is not complete unanimity of opinion as to which patient with acute myocardial infarction should be paced. We do not generally pace Mobitz Type I or Wenckebach block unless the rate is slow and associated with irritability or when there is hemodynamic compromise because of the rhythm. In general, with inferior infarctions and Wenckebach block, prognosis is good and pacing is not necessary. When anterior infarction is associated with complete heart block or Mobitz Type II second degree block, we always pace. Prognosis is of course poor, and statistical analysis is not sensitive enough in most cases to say whether or not patients are actually saved or survival is increased by pacing, but we believe it is. The more controversial problem complicating acute myocardial infarction is that of bifasicular block with right bundle branch block and left anterior fascicle block or left bundle branch block. If bifascicular block is newly developed with acute myocardial infarction, we usually do pass a temporary wire. The one caveat is that occasionally there may be a tachycardia related left bundle branch block with myocardial infarction. Such a rate-related left bundle branch block, particularly with rates above 110 per minute, often do not require pacing because the block is functional and not severe.

Atrial pacing (Fig. 1), especially in the CCU setting, is more physiologic than ventricular pacing (in the absence of heart block), and it is worth emphasizing that hemodynamics are better with atrial pacing. This technique should be used for temporary pacing if possible. A successful use of the technique is in atrial flutter converted by rapid atrial pacing at a rate above the atrial flutter rate. In

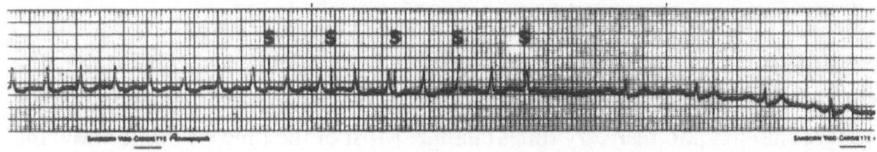

Figure 1. Conversion of atrial tachycardia to sinus rhythm by atrial pacing(s). The arrhythmia is 'interrupted' by the atrial pacing. S denotes pacemaker stimulus.

general, one usually needs overdrive pacing to convert flutter, not interruption pacing. Another use is in supraventricular tachycardia, treated by single or multiple atrial stimuli in bursts. This is the interruption type of pacing. Supraventricular tachycardia associated with the Wolf-Parkinson-White Syndrome is often well treated by either atrial or ventricular pacing, usually only a few stimuli being necessary to terminate the arrhythmia. Ventricular tachycardia also frequently can be terminated by pacing the ventricle. A re-entry ventricular tachycardia also frequently can be terminated by pacing the ventricle. A re-entry ventricular tachycardia usually can be stopped by random pacing of the right ventricle at a rate slower than the tachycardia, but occasionally overdrive pacing, faster than the tachycardia, is necessary. There have also been instances of overdriving a ventricular tachycardia by the use of atrial pacing. Ventricular pacing in the presence of ventricular tachycardia does run the risk of inducing ventricular fibrillation, and so probably should be reserved for cases of recurrent ventricular tachycardia, which would otherwise require repeated D.C. countershocks.

A less common use of rapid atrial stimulation is suppression of a supraventricular tachycardia by induction of atrial fibrillation. Sustained atrial pacing at a rate of 400-600 will either induce atrial fibrillation or pace the atria at a rate equivalent to atrial fibrillation. In either case, the ventricular rate associated with fibrillation (or its equivalent) is less than the ventricular rate associated with the supraventricular tachycardia. Such tachyarrhythmias can be suppressed and controlled by this technique for hours or days.

There are virtually no limits to arrhythmia control by pacing. The ideal place and time for pacing control of arrhythmias is in the post operative patient. Ideally we would have temporary, atrial and ventricular leads on every post cardiac surgical patient, and there are few arrhythmias which cannot be controlled with pacing. There are several mechanisms of overdrive pacing. One of these mechanisms is that at increased rates there is a narrowing of the zone of vulnerability of the heart, or decreased temporal dispersion. There is also suppression of the autonomous foci which exist in pacing tissue throughout the heart. Perhaps there is elevation of the fibrillation threshold, although in fact, the faster one paces the heart, the lower is the fibrillation threshold in many cases, especially with myocardial infarction. Lastly, pacing at a faster rate may produce slow or blocked conduction through the pathway leading to re-entry. Regardless, in overdrive pacing, something is being changed. When the rate changes, the conduction velocity through the various parts of the conduction system changes and recovery times change. Most of the time we don't know the exact mechanism operative in treating arrhythmias, but it is rational to try overdriving pacing. One can frequently produce a significant change simply by pacing the ventricle rather than having normally conducted beats.

I would like to move on to consider pacer-induced ventricular fibrillation due to a pacer stimulus falling in the vulnerable period of the preceding beat. Now this certainly is rare, and I would not in any way imply that this is a common phenomenon. It is probably extremely rare in permanent pacing, but during acute pacing, there is a phenomenon which produces a potential hazard. As shown by strength-interval curves (Fig. 2), pacing threshold at the cathode is low during electrical diastole and rises steeply during the vulnerable period when we do not want to pace. On the other hand, anodal curves show a period of time during the vulnerable period when excitation is much more easily accomplished at the anode than at the cathode. This is the underlying principle of the allegation that ventricular fibrillation is more easily produced at the anode than at the cathode. This is probably a realistic concern only in the CCU or with any acute cardiac condition, e.g. ischemia. Chronic electrodes do not as a rule show this anodal dip, which is present with acute electrodes. Studies have shown that ventricular fibrillation thresholds are lower when an anode is part of the pacing system, either through unipolar anodal stimulation, or bipolar stimulation (which includes anodal stimulation).

This led me to think that what we really need is unipolar temporary pacing.

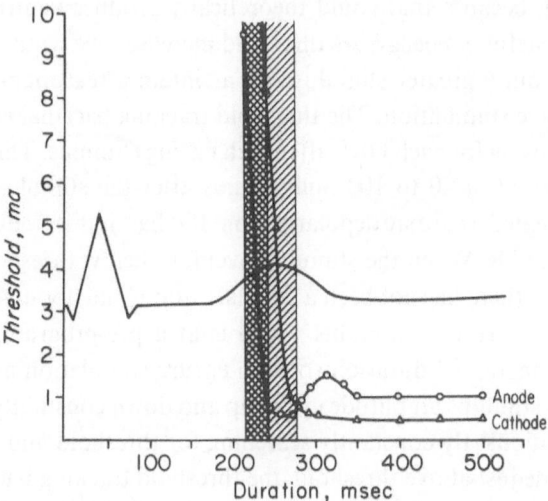

Figure 2. Anodal and cathodal strength-interval curves. During the vulnerable period the excitation threshold is lower at the anode.

Now, the ordinary method of temporary pacing is to use a bipolar catheter in which there is a cathode and an anode. My initial idea was simply to have one electrode (anode) displaced proximally on the catheter. Dr. Parsonnet told me at the beginning that I would be called at night because of unstable pacing due to this configuration. Indeed, this did happen. It's an old wives tale in pacing that unipolar catheters must be absolutely properly placed against the endocardium to obtain stimulation, whereas bipolar catheters need not have good placement, and they will pace regardless. In fact, the active electrode must be within a very short distance of the endocardium, specifically within a few millimeters. The reason that bipolar pacing is more reliable than a single unipolar electrode is that with bipolar pacing there are two electrodes in the heart, either one of which can pace the ventricle. If, with a bipolar catheter, for some reason the cathode is displaced far enough away from the endocardium, the anode usually can still pace the heart. The solution then was to produce a unipolar pacing catheter with two electrodes a centimeter apart, both of them being cathode and with the anode displaced to a position outside the heart. In this situation at least one of the two cathodes will make contact with the endocardium and provide good pacing. With the anode outside the heart, the chance of pacer-induced ventricular fibrillation is less.

I want to mention one last methodology in pacing, which is threshold tracking. Following electrode implantation, threshold usually rises to a peak within two to ten weeks and then decreases to a stable chronic level. Ideally, when threshold is low, we would like to be pacing at a level near threshold, not 10 to 20 times the threshold level, because that could theoretically produce ventricular arrhythmias and is wasteful of energy. As threshold increases, we would like our pacemakers to put out a greater stimulus and maintain a reasonable safety factor without excessive stimulation. The threshold tracking pacemaker was designed to do this by sensing for each QRS after each pacing stimulus. This device senses during the interval of 40 to 100 milliseconds after the stimulus to see if that stimulus has created a cardiac depolarization. If it has, it then reduces the output of the next stimulus. When the stimulus level falls below threshold, the instrument senses that there has not been a depolarization, and about 40 milliseconds later introduces a second stimulus which is at a pre-programmed increased amplitude and increased duration so as to ensure stimulation and depolarization. Then, the stimulus amplitude cycles up and down constantly searching for threshold variations. By constantly searching for threshold and setting the stimulus amplitude just above threshold, the threshold tracking pacemaker maintains pacer output above threshold at all times but avoids stimulation at amplitudes far above threshold. This device is still investigational and is exceedingly complex electronically, and frankly not all problems have been solved by any means. Reliable function requires absolutely perfect sensing, which is the technical limitation to date. Hopefully this device will also lead to other methods of improved pacing.

ENGINEERING CONCEPTS – HYBRID, HERMETIC, CMOS, PROGRAMMABILITY

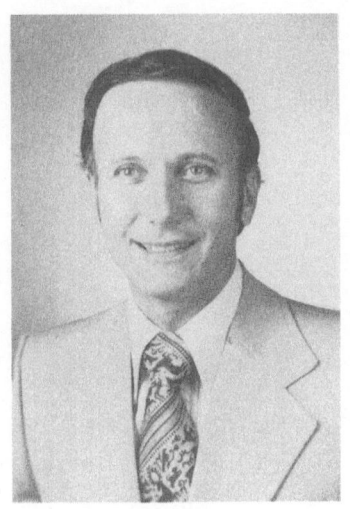

David L. Bowers, BSEE, received his degree in Electronic Engineering from California State Polytechnic University in 1960 and continues to pursue an active graduate program in the areas of biomedical engineering, cardiac physiology and creative management. From 1960 to 1972 he was a pacemaker development engineer at the General Electric Company, Medical Systems, Milwaukee. From 1972 to the present he has been an independent technical consultant in the field of medical electronics and micropower systems, specializing in cardiac pacemaker development. He is actively involved in medical research projects, investigating new concepts in applied stimulation and physiologic sensing. He is a member of IEEE and AAMI.

ENGINEERING CONCEPTS – HYBRID, HERMETIC, CMOS, PROGRAMMABILITY

DAVID L. BOWERS, BSEE

New terms and concepts are being used today to describe new and improved pacemaker devices. Many of the terms are not medical terms, but technical expressions used to indicate significant improvements in pacemaker design. This paper will attempt to identify and define some of these new terms as they relate to specific parts in a pacemaker system.

Figure 1 illustrates the basic parts comprising a pacemaker system. Figure 2

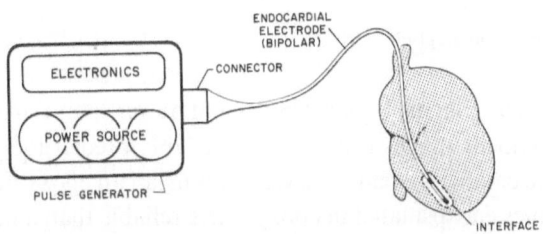

Figure 1. Pacemaker system.

diagrammatically shows how the various parts interact in a system structure. There are interactions between the electronics and power source, the electronics and conductors, and the termination of those conductors with the heart.

Todays pacemaker device could be described in the following terms:

A HERMETIC SEALED LITHIUM PACEMAKER CONTAINING HYBRID CMOS ELECTRONICS

To understand each descriptive term in the above statement, each term will be defined and related to the appropriate part in the overall pacemaker system (see (Figure 2).

The term *HERMETIC SEALED* refers to the complete pulse generative package containing the electronics and power source. A hermetic sealed package is defined as a gas-tight as well as a fluid-tight package or container preventing the controlled environment inside the package from being altered by a gas or fluid

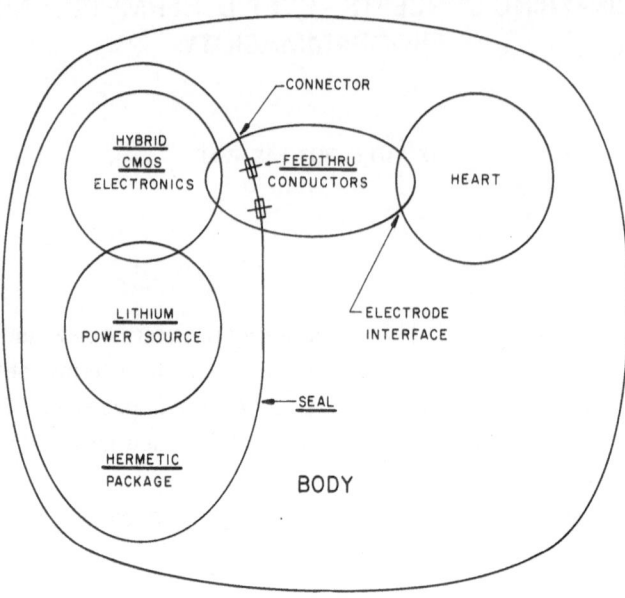

Figure 2. System interaction diagram.

outside environment. Placing the electronics and power source in a controlled or regulated environment makes it possible to reliably predict long-term performance for the pacemaker system. This does not mean an epoxy pulse generator with the electronics encapsulated in epoxy is less reliable than a hermetic sealed device, but it does mean it is more difficult to project and establish long-term performance characteristics for an epoxy device. It is also known that an epoxy device depends heavily on previous design experience and careful control of certain manufacturing processes. Therefore, a hermetic sealed pulse generator provides the best operating condition for the pacemaker system to reliably achieve its projected longevity, which means in terms of years a 5 to 10 year life expectation for present designed systems and a 10 to 20 year projection for future devices. Another advantage for the hermetic controlled environment is it makes possible the use of advanced electronic circuits such as thick-film hybrids and special semi-conductor devices which were impossible to use in an epoxy encapsulated device. If the package is to remain hermetic and stable over a 10 to 20 year period, the package originally has to be properly designed to be hermetic as well as initially tested to establish the level of hermeticity. There are various methods used to test for hermeticity, but the important criteria is to determine the total leak-rate for the package.

A technical guideline for leak-rate based on the helium leak test procedure is a leak-rate less than 1×10^{-7} standard cubic centimeters of helium per second per atmosphere. Yes, it is a very low leak-rate but necessary if the pacemaker is to retain its controlled environment over a 10 to 20 year operating life.

The next term in the descriptive statement is *LITHIUM*.This term refers to the type of power source used in the pulse generator. No attempt will be made in this paper to describe the lithium power source because it is discussed in a previous paper. I should say the lithium battery has been accepted as a long-term power source for pacemaker application.

The following two terms *HYBRID* and *CMOS* are associated with the electronics. The *HYBRID* term indicates the type of circuit construction and *CMOS* designates the type of semiconductor device used in an electronic system. A hybrid circuit can be defined as a circuit structure which combines various technologies to form a complete electronic circuit. For example, in hybrid construction thick-film technology is used to make circuit resistors combined with semiconductor technology to form active devices like transistors. This combination of technologies to form a hybrid circuit is an effective technique in the construction of sophisticated, lower current drain electronics such as used in a pacemaker.

The term *CMOS* is more difficult to define in simple technical terms. It is a special type of semiconductor transistor used in low current battery powered equipment and therefore is especially suited for pacemaker application. What do the letters C-M-O-S represent? The letters *CMOS* are derived from the first letter of each word in the following statement; Complementary Metal Oxide Semiconductor. The *CMOS* principal is based on a complementary two-transistor design with the transistors connected in series, having always one transistor in the off or non-conducting state. The only time the device consumes power is when both transistors switch from one state to another but remain complementary; one on and the other off. Because the switching time is very rapid (less than one micro-second), the power or current loss during switching is low.

Another term used to describe pacemaker function is 'Programmability.' The need for programmability in a pacemaker system is becoming increasingly necessary if the pulse generator is to be effectively matched to the needs of the heart. What are the needs of the heart? The two important needs are adequate rate and an effective stimulation response. In a programmable system the stimulus rate can be adjusted to give the best results in cardiac rhythm and function. The stimulus output from the pulse generator can be adjusted to be matched with heart threshold, usually setting the stimulus output at a selected safety margin above threshold. An important benefit derived from adapting the pulse generator to the heart is to optimize the system for the best longevity, which means the pacemaker is set to meet the special needs of the heart, not pre-set at a high and worst-case operating limit. Therefore, if the system performance is based on heart need, such as a low threshold value and minimum stimulus rate, pacemaker longevity will be optimized.

The next question is, how does a programmable system function? Figure 3 illustrates the main parts of the programmable system showing the external control interfacing with the implanted pulse generator. The purpose of the external control is to manually select the desired operating parameters for the pacemaker system and transmit this information to the pulse generator. Precautions must be taken to prevent pulse generator operation from being indiscriminately influenced by external interference. Before the external control can influence the pulse generator, the generator must be conditioned or unlocked to receive the control signals.

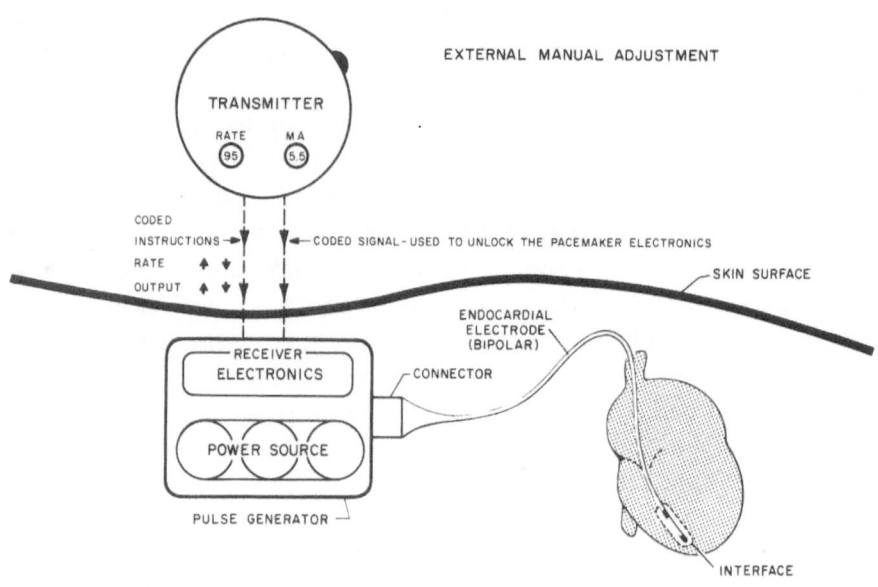

Figure 3. How does a programmable system function?

One method used to unlock the pulse generator is to send a coded signal or pattern which will prepare the electronic circuit for a new set of operating instructions. After the unlocking procedure, coded instructions are transmitted and processed in the pacemaker electronics, setting specific generator parameters to correspond with the external selected values. A disadvantage using a manual programmable system is the operating success of the pacemaker system is solely dependent on the proper selection of the parameters, i.e. rate and output.

Once the system has been set, any change in either pulse generator function or the physiological state of the heart will *not* cause a corresponding change in the preset parameter values.

A potential emergency situation could occur if the parameters were set at a minimum or marginal level. For example, exit block can occur in the case where the stimulus output was set too low and heart threshold level increased above the set value.

In my opinion, the future pacemaker system will automatically adjust and regulate pacemaker function to meet heart needs and therefore prevent improper setting of pacemaker parameters. Figure 4 illustrates how a self-regulating pacemaker will function. Information will be received from the heart and used to determine proper heart rate and threshold. After processing this information, the pacemaker output will be adjusted automatically to provide the best heart rate based on physiological need, and stimulus output level set at the appropriate value above heart threshold.

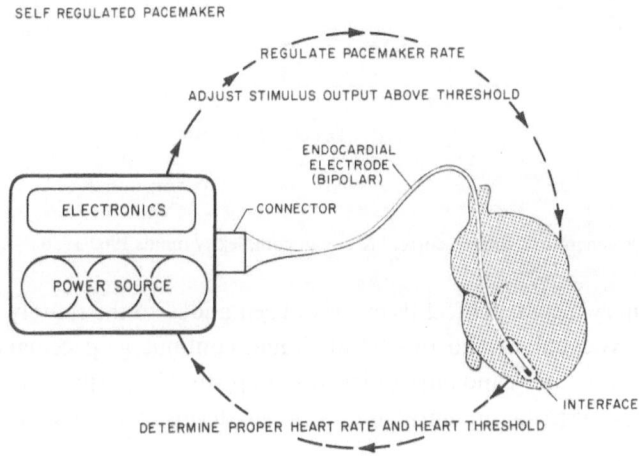

Figure 4. A future pacemaker system.

Pacemaker technical evolution since the early 1960s has progressed from a very simple electronic circuit to a sophisticated programmable system of today. This trend will continue and possibly accelerate if the self regulated pacemaker becomes a reality. To illustrate this trend pattern, Figure 5 displays a 16-year trend and a 4-year projection for circuit complexity given in component count and total current utilization from the power source. One might expect when circuit complexity increases, current drain would also increase. Instead, circuit design improvements along with technological breakthroughs has increased circuit efficiency causing a decrease in source current. Future projections indicate this decrease current trend will continue even if circuit complexity accelerates with a component count exceeding 1000 by 1980.

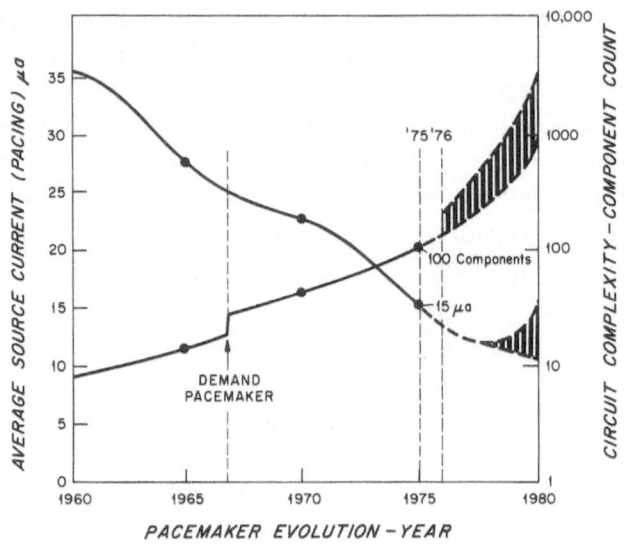

Figure 5. Pulse generator – Source current & circuit complexity trends 1960-1980.

In summary, new technical terms have been added to the rapidly expanding pacemaker vocabulary and this trend should continue as pacemaker systems become more complex and physiologically adaptive. The purpose of this paper is to define and describe presently used technical terms as well as answering this specific question:

What is a programmable hermetic sealed lithium pacemaker containing thick-film hybrid CMOS electronics?

THE IDEAL PACEMAKER

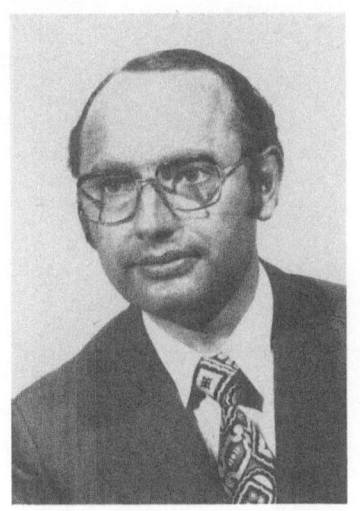

Dr. Werner Irnich received his background in electrical engineering at the Rhine Westphalian Technische Hochschule in Aachen between 1955-1960 and worked thereafter within the Department of Theoretical Electrical Engineering until 1968 when he received his doctorate for investigations of noninvasive blood pressure recording techniques. From 1968 to the present he has been associated with the medical faculty with his main field of interest and teaching involving the application of electronic engineering to diagnosis and therapy. He is the author of two books and many publications dealing with cardiac stimulation and electronics in medicine.

THE IDEAL PACEMAKER

WERNER IRNICH, PH.D.

Introduction

It is now eighteen years since the first pacemaker implantation in a human was performed in October 1958 by Elmquist and Senning. It was a rechargeable, fixed rate pacemaker which, however, only functioned for a short time. In 1963, Nathan and coworkers (12) introduced the P-wave synchronized ventricular pacemaker which was the optimal solution for patients with AV block (fig. 1b). The so called 'demand' pacemaker seems to have several inventors (5, 13). Its idea originated between 1963 and 1965. In 1966 Donato and Denoth developed the standby version, the so called R-triggered pacemaker, which has the same ability as has the demand type, namely to subordinate the pacemaker's rhythm to spontaneous beats of the heart (fig. 1a). Although the standby pacemaker is

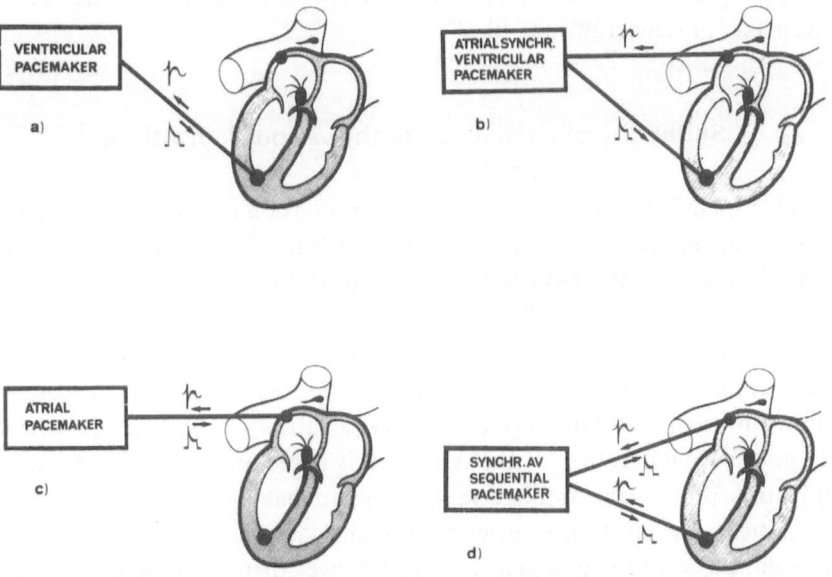

Figure 1. The various pacemaker types.

rather insensitive to interference (9), its application was reduced for two reasons:

(1) It was said to be dangerous in cases with frequent ectopic beats, and

(2) Its current consumption was normally higher than that of a demand pacemaker.

Both arguments were probably over estimated since in practice, both types are similar in behavior and longevity. For several years, the synchronized pacemaker has also been used as an atrial stimulating device (fig. 1c). Its use is restricted to few clinics which are able to anchor atrial electrodes.

At present the most complex stimulating system is the AV sequential pacemaker introduced by Berkovits in 1969 (2). This four electrode (double bipolar leads) pacemaker with two coupled channels is of the demand type with respect to the ventricular channel. The atrial channel is insensitive to atrial spontaneous beats but controlled by the ventricular channel.

A universal double channel pacemaker system which is synchronized by the atrium and also by the ventricle (fig. 1d), was proposed by us in 1975 (7). As will be shown later, it is comprised of all known types of pacemakers, but also has additional features.

The reasons why such sophisticated pacemakers are only used in such small numbers are based on the experience of the last eighteen years: excessive size, short-life, high failure rates, and difficulties with anchoring of the atrial electrodes. The physiological advantages of these systems seem to be overwhelmed by technological disadvantages which, in the future, may surely be overcome. Our problem today is, therefore, to try to answer the question, 'What will the pacemaker of tomorrow look like?'

Suitability of pacemaker to the various indications

In Table 1 a list of indications for pacemaker insertion at our clinic is given for two different intervals. It is notable that Group 2 (atrial dysrhythmias) increased from 15 percent in the 1969-1972 interval to 33.7 percent in 1973-1975. This represents a change in the indication for the implantation of a pacemaker system from a purely lifesaving to a life improving therapy.

The optimal stimulation systems for these various indications are proposed as follows: In second or third degree AV block, an atrial synchronized ventricular pacemaker would be best. If the AV block is combined with atrial flutter or fibrillation, present synchronized ventricular pacemakers would be adequate. In intermittent AV block, a ventricular demand pacemaker is applicable if the quiescent phase of the pacemaker is much longer than the stimulating phase. Otherwise a treatment as in sustained AV block would be more efficient.

In atrial bradycardia a synchronized atrial pacemaker would be the best so-

	1969-1972	1973-1975	OPTIMAL TREATMENT
NUMBER OF CASES	228	280	
GROUP 1	71.6%	59.3%	
BRADYCARDIA DUE TO A-V BLOCK			
1.1 2°+ 3° A-V BLOCK	64.8%	36.8%	ATRIAL SYNCH. V. PM
1.2 BRADYCARDIA c̄ ATRIAL FLUTTER OR FIBRILLATION · · · · · ·	4.4%	15.9%	SYNCH. V. PM
1.3 INTERMITTENT A-V BLOCK	2.4%	6.6%	VENTRIC. DEMAND PM
GROUP 2	15.0%	33.7%	
ATRIAL DYSRHYTHMIAS			
2.1 SINUS BRADYCARDIA (SUSTAINED) . .		22.0%	SYNCH. ATRIAL PM
2.2 SINUS BRADYCARDIA (INTERMITTENT)		5.1%	DEMAND ATRIAL PM
2.3 CAROTID SINUS SYNDROME		6.6%	DEMAND ATRIAL PM
GROUP 3			
COMBINATIONS OF GROUP 1 + 2	13.4%	7.0%	SYNCH. A-V SEQUENT PM

Table 1. Indications for pacemaker implantation.

lution. If it is intermittent, an atrial or a ventricular demand pacemaker is adequate. If the combination of an AV block together with an atrial bradycardia is given, an AV sequential pacemaker with synchronization by the atrium and the ventricle would be desirable.

If the distribution of the various pacemaker types is analyzed on the basis of the indication list of 1973-1975 and assuming optimal treatment, the following results are obtained (Table 2). The atrial synchronized ventricular pacemaker would range at the first place with 37 percent. It is followed by the ventricular synchronized pacemaker (our today's demand or standby pacemaker) with 28 percent and the AV sequential pacemaker with 18 percent. This 18 percent includes in addition to Group 3 (Table 1) half of all atrial bradycardias. This seems to be reasonable due to the uncertainty of the AV conduction in an already injured heart. The synchronized atrial pacemaker would reach 17 percent. In

Table 2. Distribution of the various pacemaker types.

	optimal	real 1975*
1. Atrial synchronixed ventricular PM	37%	0.88%
2. Synchronized ventricular PM (demand or stand-by)	28%	92.3%
3. Atrial – ventricular sequential PM**	18%	0.02%
4. Synchronized atrial PM (demand or stand-by)	17%	1%
5. Fixed rate PM	—	5.7%

* Worldwide estimation from the data presented in Tokyo 1976.
** If half of all atrial bradycardias are treated by SA sequential PM.

reality the situation is quite different (Table 2) (1). The ventricular pacemakers, synchronized or fixed rate, are dominating with 98 percent. All other types are insignificant and only limited to few specialized clinics.

The incidence of ectopic beats is rather high in pacemaker patients. We found only about 5 percent of our patients to be free of any ectopic beats (11), so the fixed rate pacemaker has to be excluded from the list of optimal treatments.

The problem of anchoring atrial electrodes

Up to now, no electrode has been able to be anchored within the atrium with the ease and the low complication rate of the transvenous ventricular electrode. This is perhaps one of today's most important and outstanding problems, as was demonstrated at the last pacemaker symposium in Tokyo 1976 (1). Three papers concerning this problem (Timmis et al., Toga et al., Bisping et al.) were officially presented and two further comments arose from the audience during the electrode session. Nearly all of the proposed electrodes were capable of being anchored within the atrium in some manner. Our contribution to this problem started in 1971, (3, 8, 10), yielding a troublefree electrode which, after a three year evaluation period, has been implanted in more than 1000 cases, about 50 of them within the atrium. Figure 2 and Figure 3 show the principle. During the insertion phase the hooks are held within a hollow cylinder which forms the tip (a). Having found a favourable position, the hooks spring out by their own elasticity when pushed slightly forward by a stylet (b). The electrode is covered with silicone rubber over the total length of the cylinder so that only the front side forms an electric contact with the heart. For better penetration the hooks are sharpened. With a J-shaped stylet, it is possible, without major difficulties, to anchor it within the appendage of the right atrium. This procedure may be simplified in the

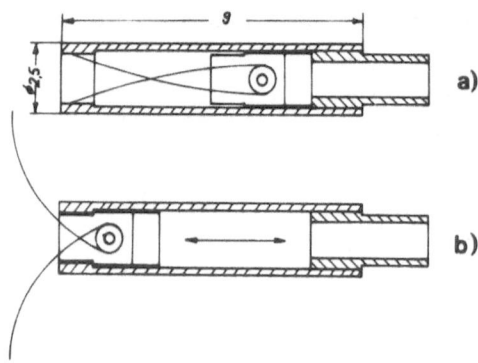

Figure 2. Principle of the hooking electrode.

future by a more flexible multiple wire lead which will also be more durable. With the availability of a simple and routinely applicable atrial electrode, future pacemaker therapy will surely be revolutionized.

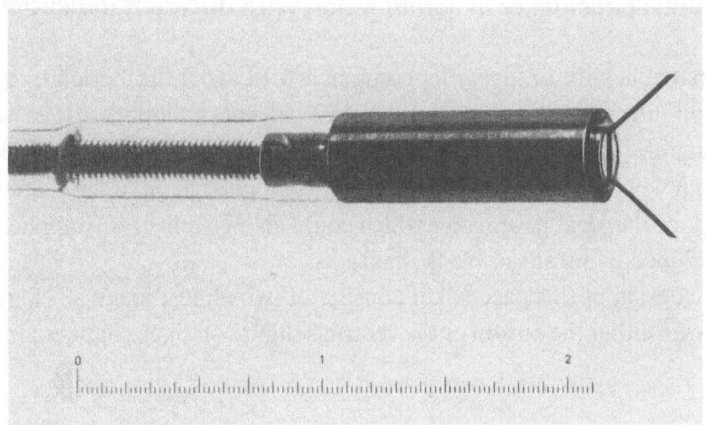

Figure 3. Photograph of the hooking electrode (scale in cm).

Energy requirement in sophisticated pacemaker systems

The use of more sophisticated circuitry together with higher frequencies results in higher current consumption and consequently in a reduction of generator lifetime. But with present electronic system design, lifetime may be more than 10 years even in double channel pacemaker systems. This may be proved by the following calculation (6). With a 10 mm^2-electrode and a pulse width of 0.5 ms a mean current of about 4µA at a frequency of 70 min^{-1} is going to the heart. If we assume the frequency of the sophisticated system to be higher, for instance 100 min^{-1}, the current consumption is increased to 100/70 times 4 µA = 5.7 µA. Together with the current consumption of the electronic circuitry which lies in the order of 8 µA or less in pacemakers with discrete elements and which goes down below 2 µA with hybrid CMOS technology, the sum of all currents lies between 7.5 and 13.7 µA. Assuming a double channel pacemaker system with stimulation of both atrium and ventricle with a current consumption of 15 µA and a desired lifetime of 10 years, the capacity of a lithium battery has to be:

$$Q = 2 \cdot 15 \text{ µA} \cdot 10 \text{ years} = 2.63 \text{ Ah}$$

(The factor 2 is necessary because of voltage doubling with lithium batteries).

A capacity of 3.3 to 3.8 Ah is now available so that energy is no longer the limiting factor. It should be pointed out that there is no atrial synchronized ventricular pacemaker available with lithium batteries today.

The universal pacemaker in combination with different indications

Except in patients with bradycardia combined with atrial fibrillation or atrial flutter and in intermittent AV block (about 23 percent of all patients) in which today's available demand pacemakers are entirely adequate, an improved pace-maker design would be desirable which could be applied in all other diagnoses. The concept of the ideal pacemaker which could also be universally applicable, will be developed by means of block diagrams.

The basic design of this pacemaker consists of two almost identical channels connected with either the atrium or the ventricle (figure 4). Each channel consists of:

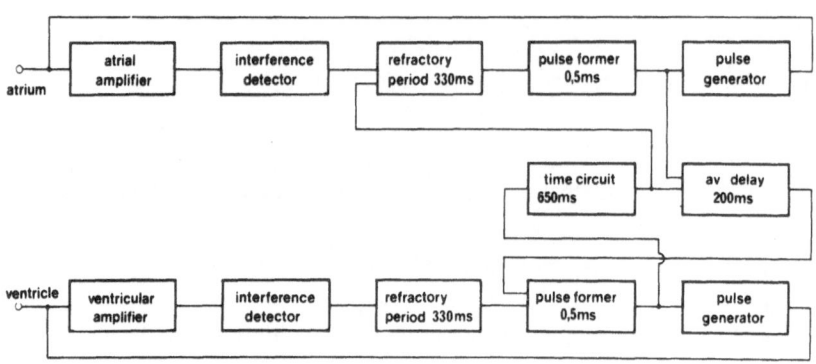

Figure 4. The universal pacemaker.

1. Amplifier
2. Filtering and interference detecting device
3. Refractory period device
4. Pulse former, for the pulse width
5. Pulse generator

The basic frequency of both channels is determined by the timing circuit which is followed by the AV delay device. Only the ventricular channel is capable of synchronizing the timing circuit, which acts directly upon the atrium but with a delay on the ventricular channel. The behavior of the total circuitry in association with various cardiac defects will be discussed in more details by demonstrating four different cases.

1. AV Block

As shown in Figure 5, the atrial signal whose frequency is assumed to be higher than the standby rate of the pacemaker, reaches the amplifier via the atrial electrode. The signal pathway is indicated in Figure 2 and in the following figures by the bold lines. Identification of the signal is undertaken at the output of the amplifier by the discrimination and filtering device. A refractory circuit delay of 330 ms ensures that the highest frequency of 180 min^{-1} cannot be exceeded. At

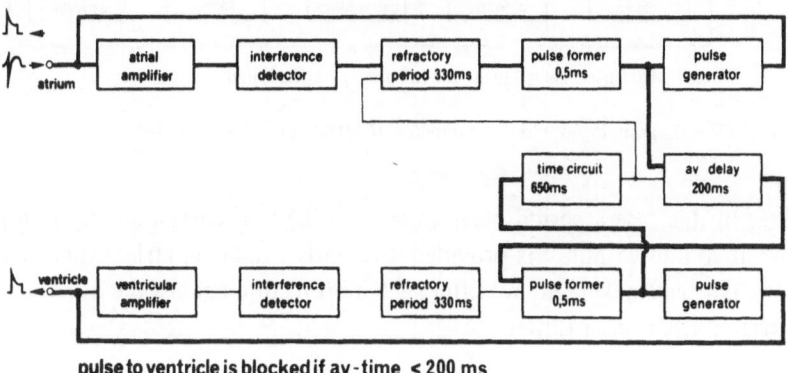

Figure 5. Flow diagram in AV block.

the same time the pulse duration is set by the pulse former, and, in our experience this should be 0.5 ms, particularly if smaller electrodes are used (8). As with the non-inhibited synchronous pacemaker, a stimulus is released to the spontaneously beating atrium. After a delay of 200 ms, the pulse former and pulse generator of the ventricular channel is triggered provided that no conducted ventricular beat has occured in the interim. Should such a spontaneous beat occur, the timing circuit together with the AV delay circuit is reset. The ventricular channel is of the demand type and spontaneous ventricular activity will inhibit the production of a stimulus.

2. AV Block Combined with Atrial Fibrillation and Atrial Flutter

During the normal atrial activity the pacemaker behaves as a normal atrial synchronized ventricular pacemaker, the only difference being that a stimulus is also released to the atrium (figure 6). If the atrial period is shorter than 330 ms (corresponding to an atrial rate of more than 180 min^{-1}), the atrial refractory period is increased to 600 ms each atrial signal which occurs after this interval causes an atrial stimulus to be released and delayed by 200 ms, a ventricular stimulus. This prevents the rate from varying between 70 and 180 min^{-1} in the case of atrial fibrillation or atrial flutter. This, therefore, protects those patients in whom atrial fibrillation or atrial flutter develops after pacemaker implan-

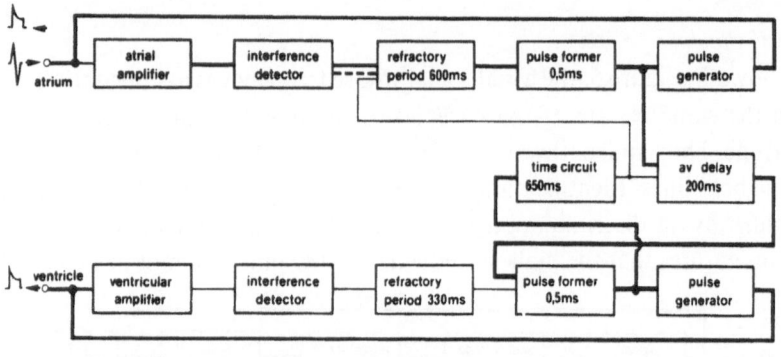

with atrial intervals < 330 ms the refractory period is increased to 600 ms

Figure 6. Flow diagram in AV block combined with atrial fibrillation or flutter.

tation. In this case a period between 800 and 850 ms corresponding to a rate between 70 and 75 min⁻¹ is provided. Presently available, atrial synchronized ventricular pacemakers do not offer such a protection against the development of atrial fibrillation or flutter.

3. *AV Block Combined with Sinus Bradycardia or SA Block*

As will be seen from Figure 7, 650 ms after the last ventricular impulse, the timing

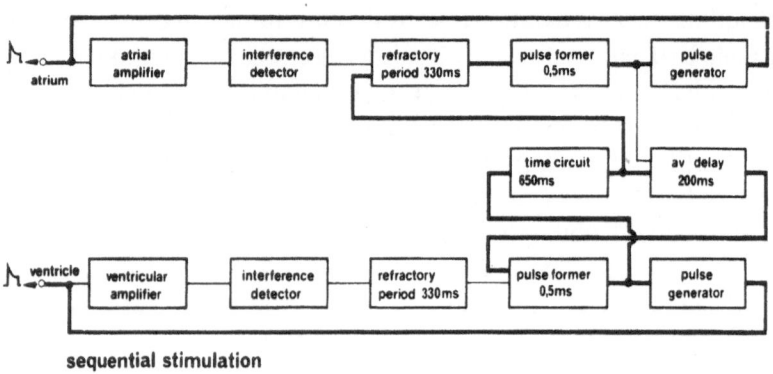

sequential stimulation

Figure 7. Flow diagram in AV block combined with sinus bradycardia or SA block.

circuit stimulates the atrium via the atrial channel and, 200 ms later, the ventricle via the ventricular channel. This provides therefore, AV sequential stimulation. A unique feature of this concept is that each ventricular ectopic beat will immediately interrupt the timing mechanism. An atrial ectopic beat will act upon the circuit via the AV delay, and the normal period without ectopic beats is 850 ms (70 min⁻¹).

4. *Sinus Bradycardia or SA Block*

The most physiological way of treating this condition is by the use of an atrial stimulator, 650 ms after the last ventricular activity by means of which the timing circuit is reset, and an impulse is released to the atrium (Figure 8). If the AV

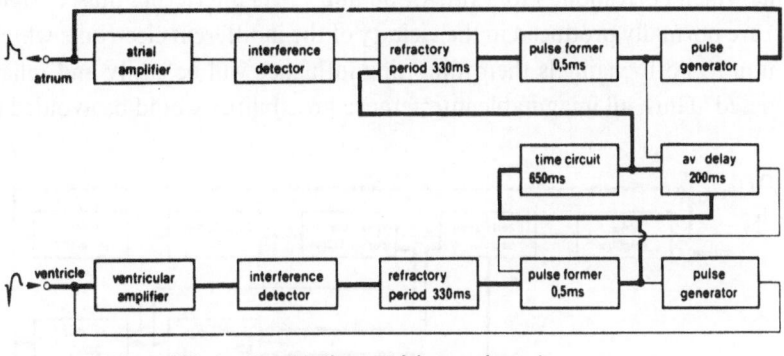

with $T_{AV} > 200$ ms, stimuli to the ventricle are released

Figure 8. Flow diagram in sinus bradycardia or SA block.

interval is greater than 200 ms, AV sequential stimulation is carried out. The period will vary, therefore, between 650 ms plus the AV interval and 850 ms, and corresponds to a rate of about 70 to 75 min^{-1}. This solution of atrial stimulation is superior to the current methods of ventricular stimulation for two reasons:

a) In our patients one could often observe that with simple ventricular stimulation coupled 'echo' beats were produced which could not always be suppressed by drugs. This is overcome by the atrial stimulation.

b) It takes into account ventricular ectopic beats. In this situation the atrium is simultaneously stimulated together with the ectopic beat, and the timing circuit as well as the AV delay circuit is reset. This function thus requires the synchronous (triggered) mode of the atrial channel. It prevents re-excitation by retrograde conduction and thus possible tachycardias. At the longest, 650 ms after the preceding ventricular ectopic beat, the next atrial excitation will take place, and 200 ms later that of the ventricle. Present AV sequential stimulators do not cover this type of arrhythmia as there is no possibility of synchronization by atrial as well as by ventricular signals.

Interference occurring at both inputs

The bifocal pacemaker, having electrodes positioned within both the atrium and the ventricle, has additional advantages of being able to recognize interference signals. Since normally atrial and ventricular signals are separated by about 150-

200 ms, signals appearing simultaneously at both inputs may be interpreted as interference (figure 9). This is very easily detected by a NAND circuit, which by reducing the interval of the timing circuit to 500 ms, increases the pacemaker frequency. In this condition the period is 500 ms plus 200 ms AV delay time or 700 ms which corresponds to a rate of 86 min^{-1}. As interfering muscle signals (emg) are normally produced in the vicinity of the indifferent electrode, which is common to both channels their inhibiting influence will be easily and reliably eliminated. Thus, all imaginable interference possibilities would be avoided (9).

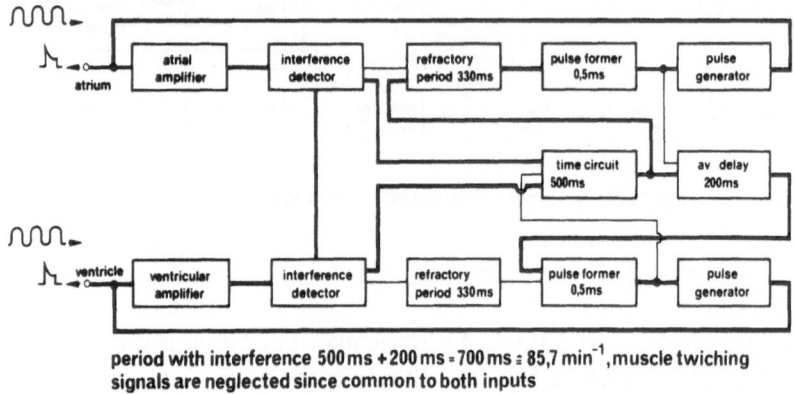

period with interference 500 ms +200 ms =700 ms ≅ 85,7 min^{-1}, muscle twiching signals are neglected since common to both inputs

Figure 9. Flow diagram with interference occurring at both inputs.

Conclusions

This concept is not a final one, but serves to demonstrate the physiological and technical possibilities, and the complexity of the interaction between the pacemaker and the heart.

The universal pacemaker would be, in most cases, a device which really restores physiological conditions. Present day pacemakers, with the exception of the P-wave synchronized ventricular one, only allow a minimal frequency. This universal pacemaker would, moreover, be helpful in some cases in which tachycardias are produced by retrograde conduction combined with ventricular ectopic beats.

In those cases with atrial bradycardia and bradycardia with atrial flutter or fibrillation (about 45 percent) a further improvement would be a frequency control according to the patient's need as proposed by Funke (4). He tried to control the heart rate by the respiratory cycle. He postulated a relationship of 4:1 between heart and respiration rate. The latter is detected by a piezoelectric transducer. It is questionable whether this method or another proposed (1) will be suitable for long term stimulation. This concept, however, should be further investigated.

One final remark should be made. Questions may arise why a concept is presented here which has not been realized so far. There are two answers:

1. The time delay between concept and introduction to the market has increasingly augmented for several important reasons. If we want to have a universal pacemaker in five years, we must begin designing it now.

2. The change from discrete element electronics to integrated hybrid technology makes it more difficult and more expensive to introduce innovations and improvements. Similar to the calculator market where you have several types with different functions but with the same integrated circuit chip in it, it is perhaps a better philosophy to have a highly sophisticated system from which all others can be derived.

Summary

In spite of considerable technical achievements in the pacemaker field, developments in this area cannot be considered complete until a universal pacemaker appropriate for all situations is available. Today, the development of such a unit is technically possible and energy sources with lifetimes in excess of ten years are available. An ideal system demands a functioning atrial electrode for both sensing and stimulation, and the benefits of this form of stimulation must be weighed against both the risks and problems involved in its applications. As far as the more complicated electrical defects of the heart are concerned, the universal pacemaker of the type discussed has advantages over conventional units, especially for those patients in whom bradycardia has been followed by tachycardia. In spite of its complexity, it can be demonstrated that the concept of the universal pacemaker is one which lends itself to a design which is highly resistant to environmental interference.

Literature

1. Abstracts of Free Communications. *Proceedings Vth International Symposium on Cardiac Pacing Tokyo 1976.* Watanabe, Y., ed. Excerpta Medica, Amsterdam 1977.
2. Berkovits, B.V., Castellanos jr. A., Lemberg, L., Bifocal demand pacing. *Circulation* Suppl. 39, 111-44, 1969.
3. Bleifeld, W-. Irnich, W., Effert, S., A new transvenous electrode with myocardial fixation. *Digest 9th Int. Conf. Med. Biol. Eng.* Melbourne 1971.
4. Funke, H.D., Ein Herzschrittmacher mit belastungsabhangiger Frequenzregulation. *Biomed. Technik* 20, 225-228, 1975.
5. Irnich, W., *Elektrotherapie des Herzens,* physiologische und biotechnische Aspekte. - Fachverlag Schiele & Schon, Berlin 1976.

6. Irnich, W., Current consumption and service life in implantable pacemakers. *Europ. J. Cardio!.* *(in press)*.

7. *Irnich, W., The Ideal Pacemaker. Proceedings of the Pacemaker Colloquium.*Norman, J. and Rickards, A. eds. Vitatron medical, Arnhem 1976.

8. Irnich, W., Engineering concepts of pacemaker electrodes. *Advances in pacemaker technology,* Schaldach, M. and Furman, S., eds. Springer, Berlin 1975.

9. Irnich, W., De Bakker, J.M.T., Bisping, H.J., Electromagnetic interference in implantable pacemakers pace (in press).

10. Irnich, W., Bleifeld, W., Effert, S., Permanente transvernose Elektrostimulation des Herzens mit einer myokardial fixierten Elektrode. *Thoraxchirurgie* 20, 440-443, 1972.

11. Merx, W., Meiselbach, K., Irnich, W., Effert, S., Are fixed-rate pacemakers indicated in patients with constant total AV Block? *Abstracts 7th Europ. Conf. Cardiol.* Amsterdam 157, 1976.

12. Nathan, D.A., Center, S., Chang-You-Wu, Keller, W., An implantable synchronous pacemaker for the longterm correction of complete heart block. *Am. J. Cardiol.* 11, 362, 1963.

13. Thalen, H.J.Th., Van den Berg, J.W., Homan van der Heide, J.N., Nieveen, J., *The Artificial Cardiac Pacemaker*, it history, development and clinical application. Royal Van Gorcum, Assen 1969, 3rd printing 1975.

DIFFERENTIAL DIAGNOSIS OF PACEMAKER SYSTEM FAILURE

J. WARREN HARTHORNE, M.D.

Differential diagnosis of pacemaker system failure

As with any new therapeutic modality, the advent of cardiac pacing in the late 1950's brought with it a whole spectrum of faulty and erratic pacemaker performance. This review of pacemaker system failure is, of necessity, an anecdotal and personalized one designed to stimulate the reader's attention toward stepwise analysis in individual cases rather than to present an exhaustive compendium of each and every sample of erratic pacemaker behaviour reported in the literature. With each passing day, previously unrecognized mechanisms of pacemaker system malfunctions are identified. The key to successful interpretation is a flexible and curious analytic approach. No attempt is made to discuss complications of pacemaker surgery other than those intrinsic to the equipment. Complications of atrial pacing are also not discussed. A pacemaker 'system', whether permanent or temporary, is comprized of three general units: the energy source, the electrode, and the electronic circuit. Just as the weakest link in the chain determines its ultimate strength, that portion of the pacemaker system with the lowest reliability determines the functional performance of the overall 'system.' For the purpose of order and organization, this presentation on the detection of pacemaker system failure will illustrate examples of aberrant function of each of these three sub-units separately plus a brief discussion of miscellaneous problems. It should be apparent to the reader that the mind is more complex than the written word and that, in practice, when faced with pacemaker system failure, one synthesizes and analyzes all of the evidence simultaneously to provide a focus on the most likely cause of the problem. Erratic pacemaker behaviour is, of course, not confined to permanent systems alone and is equally or more often a consequence of temporary pacing. In general, the nature of the problem is similar so that no attempt is made to isolate the description of each. Certain types of malfunction, although common to both forms of cardiac stimulation, tend to be more common with temporary pacing: eg. loose electrode connections, malposition of electrodes, radio-frequency interference, and sepsis.

A. *The Energy Source*

The reader is referred to Dr. Cywinski's review of pacemaker energy sources for technical information. All pacemaker systems, if functioning long enough, will show evidence of battery depletion. Conversion of the zinc components into zinc oxide, which occurs during the electrochemical process of generating energy in the standard RM1 type cell, results in loss of clarity of the cylindrical ring configuration of fresh batteries. During the early days of pacemaker follow-up clinics, serial x-rays of pulse generators were employed as a rough approximation of residual battery energy (Fig. 1). More exact methods of follow-up have

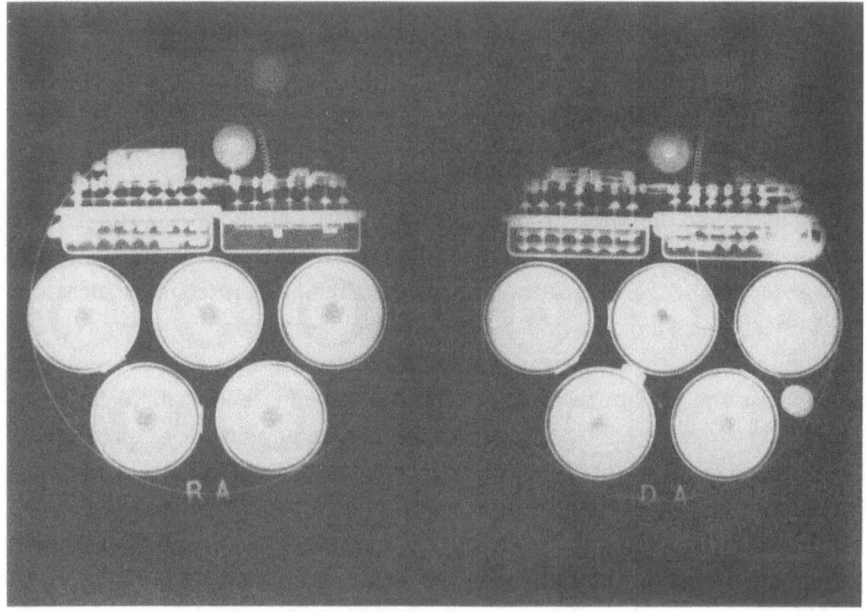

Figure 1. X-ray of fresh (left) and outdated (right) mercury zinc pacemaker. Note the loss of clarity of the internal ring configuration (Cordis omnicor series).

rendered this method obsolete. Most of the mercury zinc powered pacemaker systems are designed to show some variation of the basic stimulation rate as battery depletion developes (Fig. 2). The majority of such systems today will develop slowing of the stimulation rate. On the average the rate slows approximately 10% of the base rate as each cell depletes. Having the patient record his peripheral pulse daily may provide reassurance of the stability of pacing in those patients whose cardiac rhythm is under complete control by the pacemaker device. For patients with spontaneous escape rhythms, peripheral pulse recording will reflect whichever rhythm (i.e. paced or spontaneous) is manifest at the time and the patient must be instructed that his peripheral pulse rate should not

A.T. #003-00-42   Cordis Ectocor (#129C)

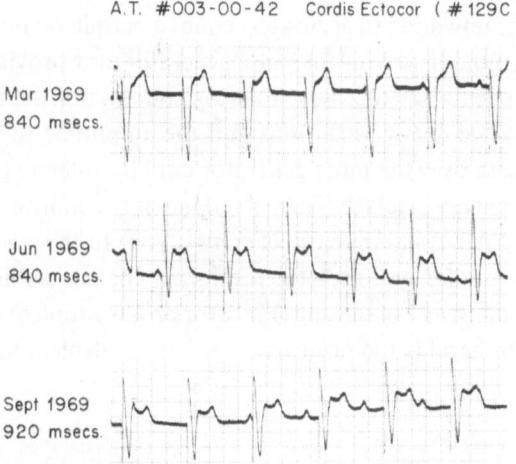

Mar 1969
840 msecs.

Jun 1969
840 msecs.

Sept 1969
920 msecs.

Figure 2. Serial strips showing decline in stimulation rate reflecting battery depletion (21 months).

fall below the escape rate of the pacemaker but can rise above it. Many physicians working in the pacemaker field prefer *not* to have patients concern themselves with daily pulse recording because of the confusion (and anxiety!) which may result when pacemaker induced and spontaneous beats coexist. For patients

MGH #003-00-42

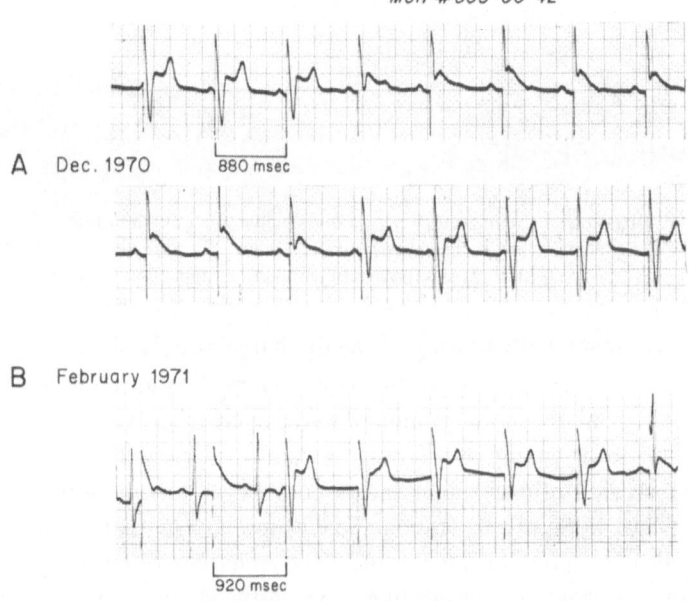

A   Dec. 1970   880 msec

B   February 1971

920 msec

Figure 3. Decline in stimulation rate plus reversion to asynchronous pacing reflecting battery depletion. (Cordis Ventricular Synchronous Ectocor Model 144G).

who prove unable or unwilling to accurately count a peripheral pulse, the use of an A.M. transistor radio held over the pulse generator may provide an acoustical pick-up of the pacing artefact which allows counting of the rate. The dial selector must be placed between stations and the amplitude turned up while rotating the radio case over the pulse generator until its antenna (usually in the back) picks up the pacing artefact. This technique only confirms emission of a pacing stimulus and not resultant cardiac contraction. In the event of a perforated, dislodged, or broken electrode the results may be misleading.

With demand systems, loss of sensing (Fig. 3) or prolongation of the refractory period (Fig. 4) often heralds the occurrence of battery depletion. This usually

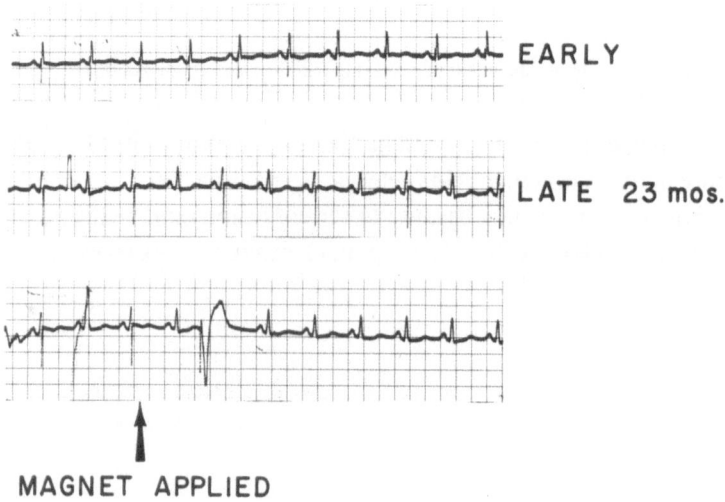

MAGNET APPLIED

Figure 4. Prolongation of the refractory period and decline in stimulation rate reflecting battery depletion (Cordis Ventricular synchronous Ectocor Model 129) Note alternate synchronization during the late recording with total cessation of function after application of magnet.

occurs in company with slowing of the discharge rate. With advanced battery depletion complete (Fig. 5) or partial (Fig. 6) loss of capture will appear.

Experience with the newer lithium powered pacemaker systems is too short to provide illustrative examples of failure mechanisms. The reader is referred to Dr. Cywinski's review of pacemaker energy sources for a discussion of the failure modes of Saft lithium cells (which show a double rate pattern) and Lithium Iodide cells (slow gradual rate decline). The rechargeable nickel cadmium systems show a variable rate according to when the system was charged. It thus becomes essential with monitoring of such patients that the stimulation rate be recorded at a fixed interval following charging. The pulse width of the pacemaker

W.S. #153-63-30   Medtronic #5841

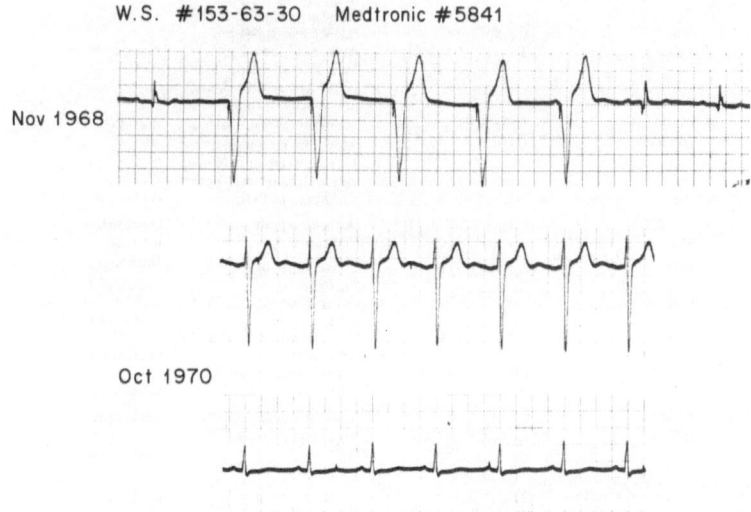

Nov 1968

Oct 1970

Admitted for "elective" generator change. Admission ECG shows
slow ineffective firing of generator.

Figure 5. Total loss of capture with slowed rate of discharge reflecting battery depletion (Medtronic Model 5841).

SUPRANORMAL CAPTURE:

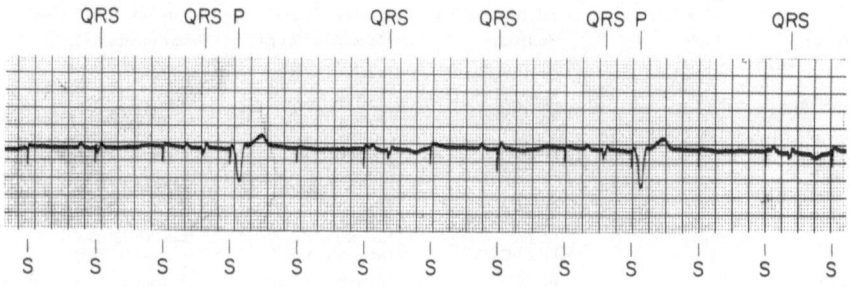

Figure 6. Intermittent capture due to battery depletion. Note that capture occurs during the supranormal phase of endogenous complexes. (S = Stimulus P = Pace).

stimulus may also fluctuate according to residual battery life (Table 1). Reduction in the amplitude of the pacemaker stimulus in the surface electrocardiogram may provide a rough approximation of waning battery reserves although accurate quantitation is difficult.

Table 1. Battery depletion: End of Life Indicators[1] (EOL)

Manufacturer	Model Number	Energy Source[2]	Stimulus Rate Change[3]	Stimulus Pulse Width Change
American Pacemaker Co	Predicta 4	Zn/HgO	Auto. rate down 2 ppm Mag. rate up 6-9 ppm Gap between auto. & mag. rate widens to 18 ppm	unchanged
	1600 series	Li I$_2$ (CRC802/23)	Auto. rate down 2 ppm Mag. rate up 6-9 ppm Gap between auto. & mag. rate widens to 18 ppm	unchanged
	8100 series (Bifocal)	LiAg$_2$CRO$_4$ (saft)	Auto. rate down 2 ppm Mag. rate up 6-9 ppm Gap between auto. & mag. rate widens from 11 ppm to 17 ppm at EOL	unchanged
Technology	DU 301 DB 301	LiI$_2$ (CRC 801/23) LiI$_2$ (CRC 801/23)	Decrease 5 ppm Decrease 5 ppm	increase[4] increase
ARCO	Li2D	LiSoCl$_2$(GTE)	Convergence of mag. & auto. rate	unchanged unchanged
	Li3D	LiSoCl$_2$(GTE)	Convergence of mag. & auto. rate	unchanged
	Li4D	LiSoCl$_2$(GTE)	Convergence of mag. & auto. rate	unchanged
	Nu5D	Plutonium (ARCO)	Convergence of mag. & auto. rate	unchanged
Biotronik	IDP84 IDP54L	Zn/HgO LiAg$_2$CRO$_4$ (saft)	Auto. rate decrease 10% Auto. rate decrease 7-10 ppm	unchanged unchanged
Cardiac Pacemakers Inc.	Maxilith 0301UD Minilith 0501UD Minilith 0502UD	LiI$_2$(WG702E) LiAg$_2$Cro$_4$(Saft) LiI$_2$(WG752)	Decrease 6 ppm Decrease 6 ppm Decrease 6 ppm	unchanged unchanged unchanged
Coratomic	L-500 C-101	LiPbI$_4$(Mallory) Plutonium (Coratomic)	Slow decline: change at 10% Decrease 5 ppm	unchanged unchanged
Cordis	Ventricor 153 Stanicor 143 Ectocor 144 Omni Ventricor 167 Omni Stanicor 162 Omniectocor 163 Lambda 190	Zn/HgO Zn/HgO Zn/HgO Zn/HgO Zn/HgO Zn/HgO LiCuS (Dupont)	Decrease 10% Decrease 10% Decrease 10% Decrease 13% Decrease 13% Decrease 13% Stable rate until EOL: change at 7% decrease	Increase up to 2.0 msecs Increase up to 2.0 msecs Increase up to 2.0 msecs Increases acc. to rate change Increases acc. to rate change Increases acc. to rate change Increases acc. to rate change
	Nuclear 184	Plutonium (Hittman)	Decrease 13%	Increases acc. to rate change
General Electric[5]	Sentry 75	Zn/HgO	Decrease of 7 ppm	unchanged
Intermedics	C-MOS-1 Interlith (Model 223)	Zn/HgO LiI$_2$ (CRC802/23)	Decrease of 3 ppm Decrease of 5 ppm	increases increases
Medcor	3-70B 3-70C (Lithicron)	Zn/HgO LiAg$_2$CrO$_3$(Saft)	Decrease of 5-6 ppm Decrease of 7 ppm	unchanged unchanged
Medtronic	5944 5945 5950 5951 5954 5955 5972 5973	Zn/HgO Zn/HgO Zn/HgO Zn/HgO Zn/HgO Zn/HgO LiI$_2$(WG742) LiI$_2$(WG742)	Decrease 7 ppm Decrease 7 ppm Decrease 7 ppm Decrease 7 ppm Decrease of 4% of programmed rate Decrease of 4% of programmed rate Decrease of 8 ppm 3 Decrease of 8 ppm 3	Increases 1 msec Increases 1 msec Increases 1 msec Increases 1 msec Increases 1.2 msec Increases 1.3 msec Increases 1.0 msec Increases 0.7 msec
Pacesetter	BD 102 100B Series L	NiCd (Rechargeable) LiI$_2$(CRC802/23)	Decrease of 10% Decrease of 10%	Decrease of 10% + inability to retain charge Increases
Starr-Edwards	8116 20S 21S	Zn/HgO LiAg$_2$CrO$_4$(saft)	Decrease 10% Decrease 11% Decrease 11%	Increase Slight Increase Slight Increase
Telectronics	120 140 150B	LiI$_2$(WG702E) LiAg$_2$CrO$_3$(Saft) LiI$_2$(WG752)	Decrease if 8-9 ppm Decrease of 8-9 ppm Decrease of 8-9 ppm	 unchanged unchanged
Vitatron	42RT 2130	Zn/HgO LiI(CRC801/23)	Auto. rate decreases 5 ppm Mag. rate decreases 6 ppm Auto. rate decreases 4 ppm Mag. rate decreases 6 ppm	 Increases 25% Increases 15%

1. The restraints of space do not allow more elaborate or complete listing of the end of life indicators of all available models. The reader is encouraged to view this table only as a guide and to check manufacturers technical brochures for details. The information listed has been confirmed by the manufacturers or their representatives.

2. Abbreviations: mag = magnetic; auto = automatic; EOL = end of life; W.G. = Wilson Greatbatch; CRC = Catalyst Research Company.

3. In many instances with lithium powered systems, gradual rate changes throughout the life of the pacemaker may be seen. The quoted EOL rate changes are often arbitrarily selected.

4. The pulse width of the American Technology pacemaker fluctuates according to the load in the automatic rate but remains fixed in the magnetic rate until EOL.

5. Ceased production 1977.

B. *The Electrode:*

Pacemaker failure due to faults in the electrode occur due to:

1. instability of the connection between the pacemaker output terminal and lead terminal
2. mechanical breaks in the continuity of the electrode somewhere between the pacemaker generator and point of impact of the electrode tip within the endocardium
3. physical dislodgement of the electrode tip out of the chamber in which stimulation is intended
4. perforation of the myocardium with entry of the electrode into the pericardial space
5. threshold rise due to local tissue reaction around the electrode-myocardial interface.

Each of these will be examined separately, but it should be emphasized that overlap often exists: e.g. threshold rise due to perforation or dislocation is probably the most common early problem with temporary or permanent transvenous systems.

1. Interruption of the connection between the pacemaker output terminal and electrode terminal is a not uncommon observation with temporary pacemakers. Part of the regular nursing care regimen in the care of such patients should include checking these terminals for physical tightness and electrode contact (Fig. 7). The electrocardiogram which results shows erratic stimulation as the

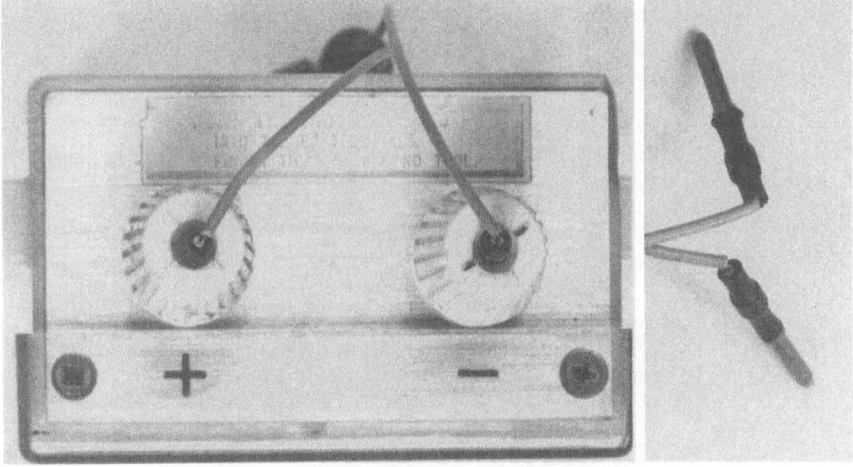

Figure 7. Photo of frayed temporary lead connector caused by patient pulling on electrode. Intermittency of contact with resultant erratic capture may ensue.

loose connection makes and breaks contact. A further source of intermittent pacing with temporary pacemakers occurs when electrode terminals are not properly insulated from each other allowing shorting out. This may occur when overlying bedclothes and linen become soaked with perspiration or other conductive liquids. Intermittency of contact is less frequently seen with permanent pacing systems but may occur when the implanting physicians fails to insert the lead terminal far enough into the pacemaker or forgets to tighten down the output terminal set screw adequately. A further cause of intermittency of capture is seen in the rare instance of a defect in the electrical weld which attaches the terminal pin of the electrode to the helical coil spring of the electrode itself (Fig. 8).

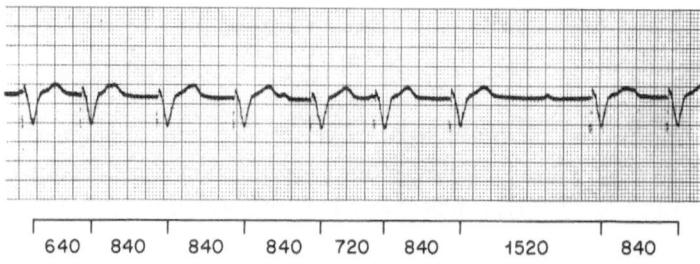

Figure 8. EKG rhythm strip showing irregular stimulation frequency due to defective electrical weld in lead terminal. (Cordis Ventricular Synchronous Ectocor Model 144G7. Dec. 1974. basic interval 840 msecs.)

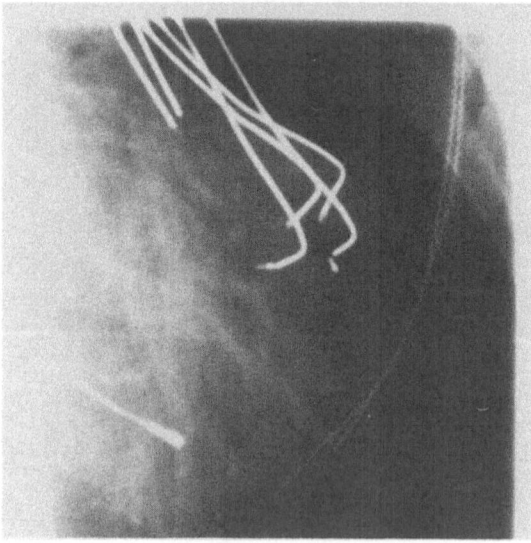

Figure 9. X-ray of epicardial electrode showing fracture of lead tip due to shear stress.

2. Mechanical breaks in the continuity of the electrode occur at points of maximum stress. This may be a shear force as with fracture of the tip of epicardial electrodes (Fig. 9) or flexion which affects myocardial electrodes where they exit from the thoracic cavity or enter the pulse generator (Fig. 10). However, one

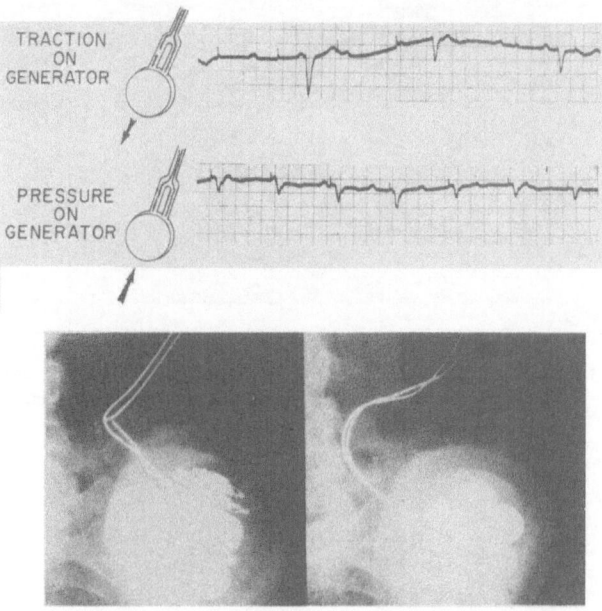

Figure 10. X-ray showing fracture of epicardial electrode at pulse generator (left) and following repair (right) Traction on the pulse generator may provide confirmation.

must be cautious to avoid over interpretation of x-rays in patients with functioning pacemakers since 'pseudo fractures' may occur (Fig. 11). With transvenous leads the breaks tend to occur at the site of anchoring sutures (which should never be used) or at the site of entry into the venous systems (Fig. 12). The electrocardiogram which results in patients with fixed rate units demonstrates erratic capture without a change in the basic stimulation rate as the fractured ends make and break contact (Fig. 13). With ventricular triggered pacemakers, premature firing of the pulse generator may be 'triggered' by the frayed ends rubbing together. X-rays intended to demonstrate lead fracture must be carefully taken and combined with fluoroscopy since a few degrees of obliquity may obscure a break due to overlap (Fig. 14).

3. Physical dislodgement of the electrode from within the heart becomes less common with increasing experience and can best be recognized by faulty capture and overpenetrated x-rays to demonstrate electrode position. Confirmation of initial lead position by predischarge chest x-rays for future comparison thus

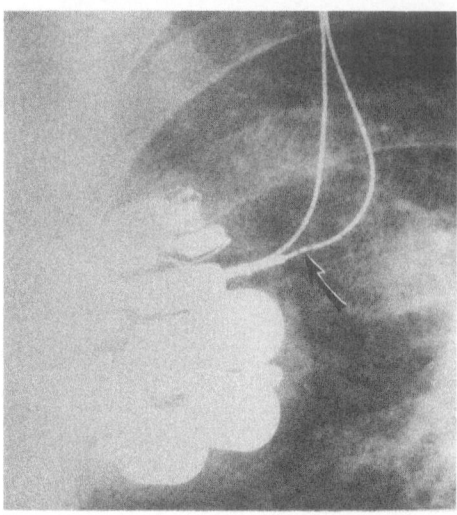

Figure 11. 'Pseudo fracture' of electrode. Medtronic bipolar electrode Model # 5816 implanted 1965. Attenuation of coil spring without fracture confirmed at subsequent generator change. Dependable function with acceptable threshold has continued for over 10 years.

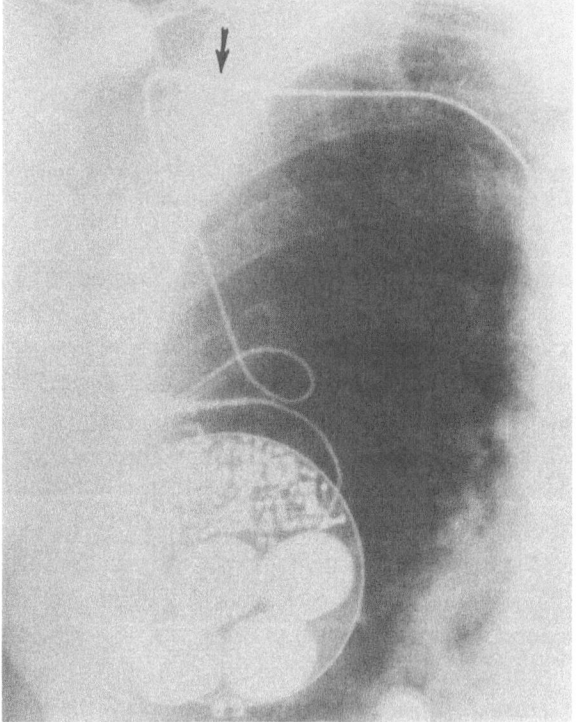

Figure 12. X-ray showing fracture of transvenous electrode at characteristic location.

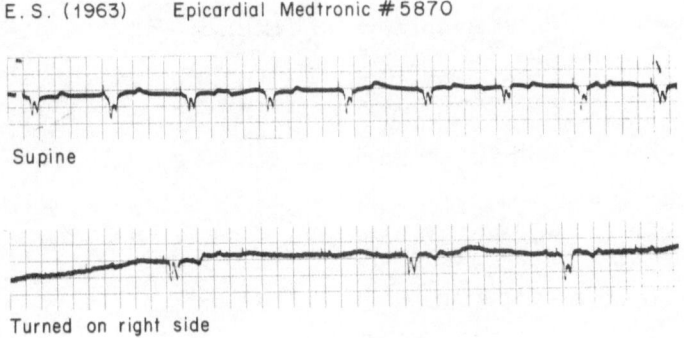

E. S. (1963)   Epicardial Medtronic #5870

Supine

Turned on right side

Figure 13. EKG showing erratic capture of pacemaker dependent upon body position – a feature which is characteristic of lead fracture.

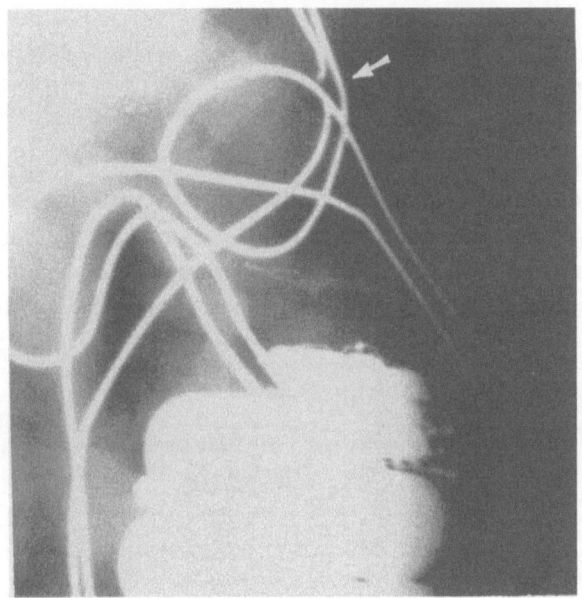

Figure 14. X-ray of epicardial lead fracture just below costal margin. A few degrees of obliquity may result in failure to identify due to overlap.

becomes very important. If the electrode recoils into the right atrium, atrial pacing may ensue and, in some instances (Fig. 15) phrenic nerve stimulation with right hemidiaphragmatic contractions results. In other instances, the electrode may advance into the pulmonary artery or recoil down the inferior vena cava. When a transvenous ventricular electrode loses its fixation but remains within the ventricular cavity, a chaotic rhythm appears with effective and ineffective

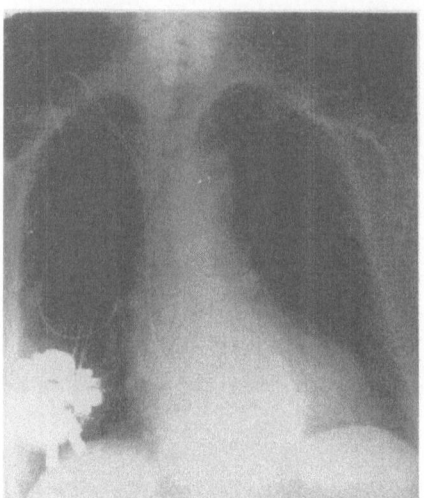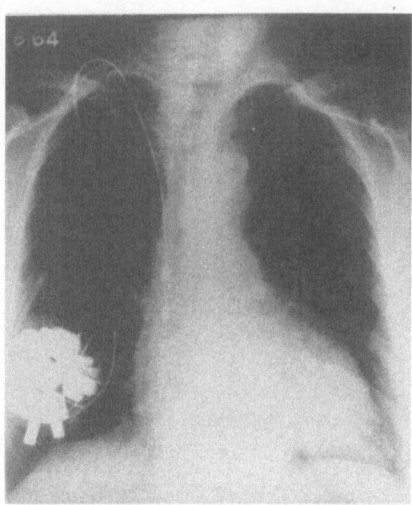

Figure 15. X-ray showing permanent transvenous pacemaker (Medtronic Model 5860) immediately following implant and 2 weeks later when pacemaker failure ensued with contraction of the diaphragm. Note that the lead tip has withdrawn to the superior vena cava adjacent to the right phrenic nerve.

stimuli interspersed with mechanically induced ventricular premature beats as the dislodged lead flails around the right ventricular cavity (Fig. 16).

4. Perforation of the myocardium is, perhaps, the commonest complication of transvenous temporary and permanent pacing and, in this author's ex-

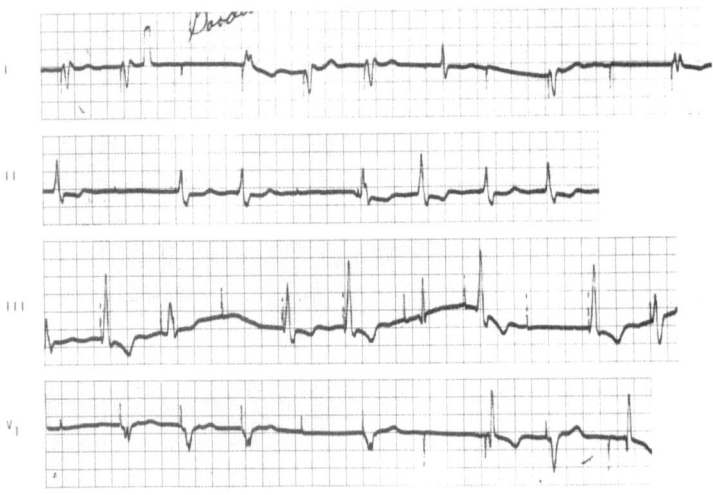

Figure 16. EKG rhythm strip in a patient with a dislodged right ventricular electrode. Note that, as the electrode flails around the ventricle a variety of complexes – some paced and non-paced and some mechanically induced are seen.

perience, is the commonest cause of failure due to a threshold rise. The occurrence of tamponade or hemodynamic embarrassment is surprizingly infrequent despite multiple perforations in the same patient but must always be anticipated. (Examples of chronic ventricular perforation with years of effective pacing are sporadically found at autopsy by most large pacemaker groups.) The usual result of perforation is erratic capture – often with preservation of normal sensing (Fig. 17) as the perforated electrode tip burrows into the epicardial fat. Complete

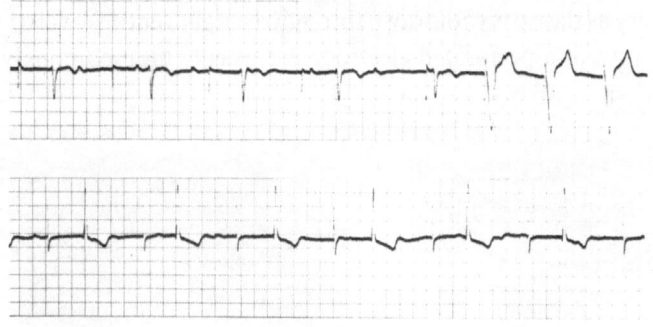

Figure 17. EKG rhythm strip of a patient with perforation of a permanent transvenous (Vitatron) electrode. Note that proper sensing of endogenous complexes continues with erratic capture plus one area of T wave sensing.

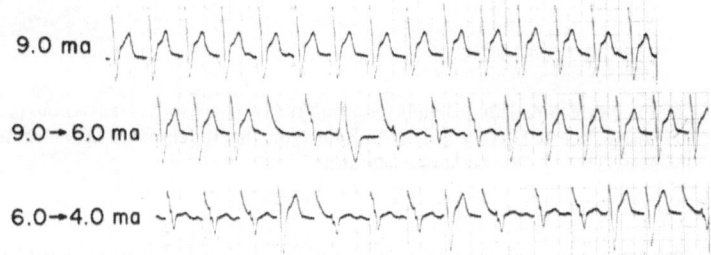

WITHDRAWAL ELECTROGRAM

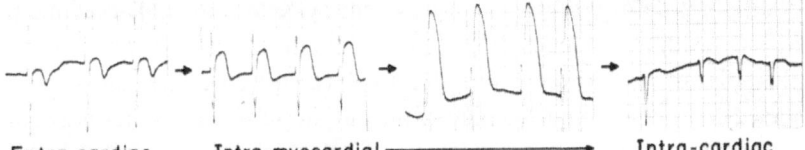

Extra-cardiac   Intra-myocardial ──────────────▶ Intra-cardiac

Figure 18. Composite EKG strips recorded during output reduction of Cordis Omnicor (model 162C) pacemaker. Note that dependable pacing continues at an output level of 9.0 ma, but becomes erratic at 6.0 ma suggesting an unsatisfactory stimulation threshold. The pullback electrogram in the lower panel confirms a current of injury as the lead is withdrawn through the right ventricular wall.

failure of capture and sensing with an x-ray which shows the electrode in seemingly acceptable position is almost pathognomonic for perforation. Rarely, on fluoroscopy, one can observe the electrode tip to project into the radiolucent epicardial fat pad. Usually, lateral chest x-rays will show the lead tip to lie in an abnormally anterior position and intercostal or left hemi-diaphragmatic contractions may ensue. If a programmable pacemaker allowing reduction of output has been employed the elevated threshold due to perforation can be demonstrated. Pullback electrograms recorded from the perforated lead will confirm a current of injury as the tip is withdrawn through the right ventricle wall (Fig. 18). Plain chest x-rays of a perforated electrode are usually disappointingly subtle (Fig. 19).

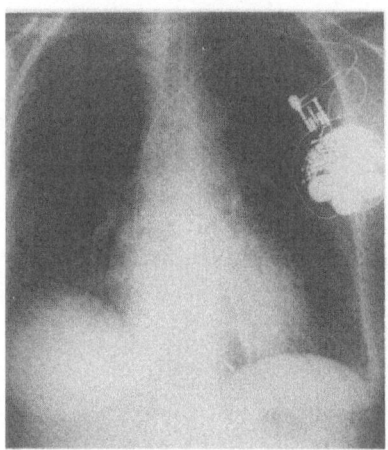 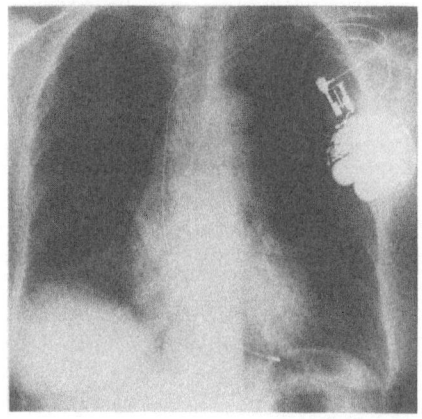

Figure 19. Chest x-rays recorded immediately following and two weeks after transvenous pacemaker insertion when failure occurred due to lead perforation. Note that the electrode tip has shifted to the left with a slight angulation at the point of perforation.

5. Threshold rise as a primary cause of early pacemaker failure is uncommon unless combined with one of the foregoing mechanisms. However, with the continuing survival of patients whose lead systems were implanted many years ago and with the diminishing pulse width of modern day pacemaker generators, examples of pacemaker failure due to elevated lead thresholds are becoming increasingly common. Matching of the output pulse width of testing equipment at the time of generator replacement to the pulse width of the device to be implanted is thus critically important. (The reader is referred to Dr. Thalen's discussion of electrodes.)

C. *The electronic circuit:*
The energy supplied by the battery and transmitted to the heart via the electrode

is modulated by the output circuit to have certain characteristic features among which are impulse frequency or rate, impulse duration or pulse width, and amplitude. At the same time, non-competitive pacemakers have a sensing circuit which is intended to detect spontaneously occuring cardiac activity so that competitive stimulation may be avoided. Without delving too deeply into the complexities of electronic technology, it is important to emphasize certain features of the sensing circuit so that misinterpretation of pacemaker function can be avoided. To avoid detection of low amplitude signals such as P waves and T waves, most sensing circuits have a sensitivity which ranges around 1.5 to 2.0 millivolts. With temporary pacemakers, this sensitivity adjustment is variable. In certain instances, the endocardial signal returning to temporary or permanent pulse generators may be of insufficient amplitude to allow detection by the sensing circuit with resultant competitive pacing (Fig. 20). Although this might appear outwardly as

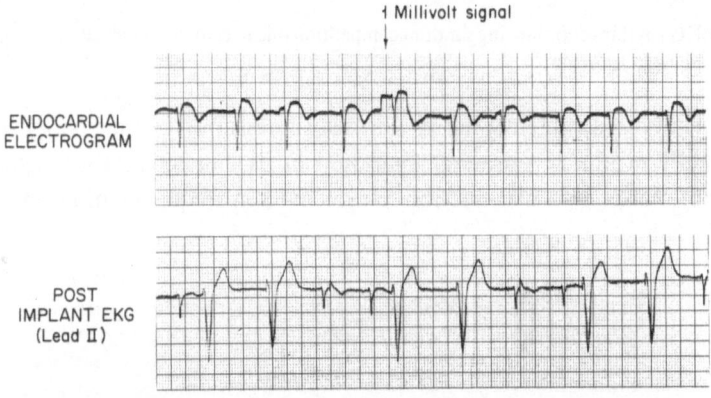

Figure 20. EKG rhythm strip showing erratic sensing; the upper strip shows the endocardial signal recorded at multiple locations throughout the right ventricle.

an electronic malfunction, the pacemaker functions exactly as designed and the problem is one of inadequate endocardial signal strength (often due to extensive prior infarction). Correction of this (infrequent) problem requires revision of the electrode position or use of a high sensitivity pacemaker. Another feature of the sensing circuit which may determine improper demand function is the frequency spectrum of the endocardial signal and its rate of rise (slew rate). Even though adequate precautions have been taken at the time of pacemaker insertion to ensure the adequacy of endocardial signal strength, subsequent evidence of failure to detect random beats of ectopic origin having sub-threshold amplitude, frequency, and slew rate may occur (Fig. 21). This is a further example of pacemaker 'malfunction' due to problems inherent in the patients cardio-vascular system. True electronic component malfunction is, fortunately, a rare event since

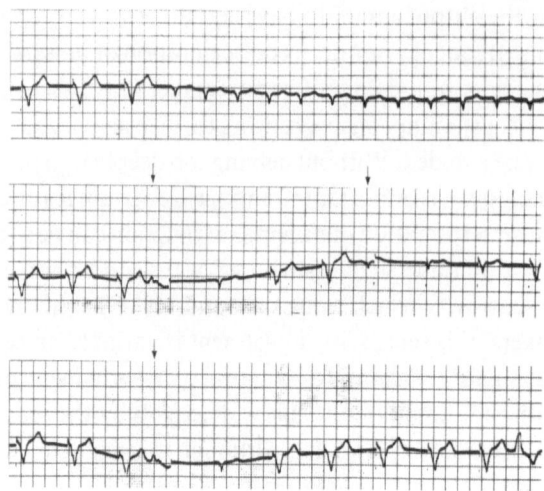

Figure 21. EKG rhythm strip showing random competition due to ectopic complexes of suboptimal amplitude, indicated by arrows.

the results are often catastrophic in contrast to depletion of the energy source which usually produces a gradual alteration in pacemaker performance. The incidence of component malfunction has declined in frequency in recent years

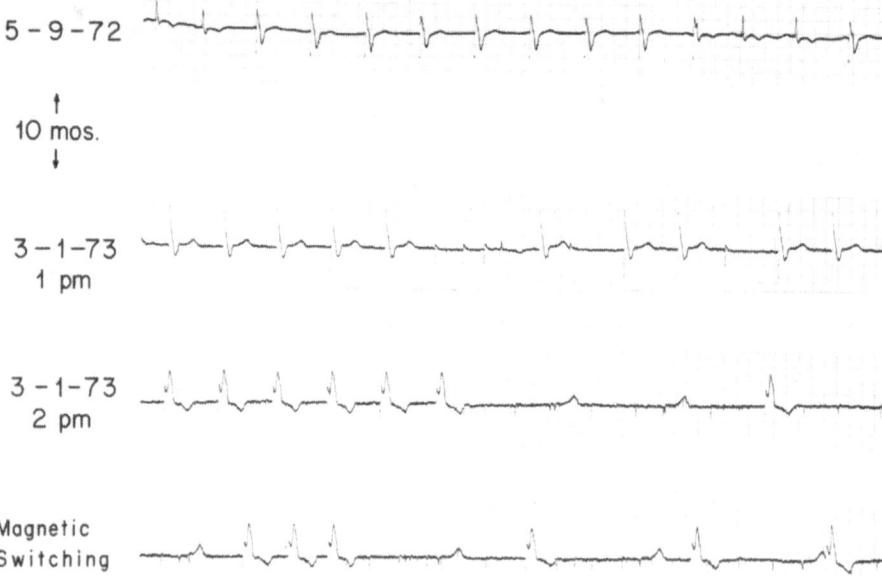

Figure 22. EKG rhythm strip of erratic pacemaker function due to component malfunction (Starr Edwards, Model 8114).

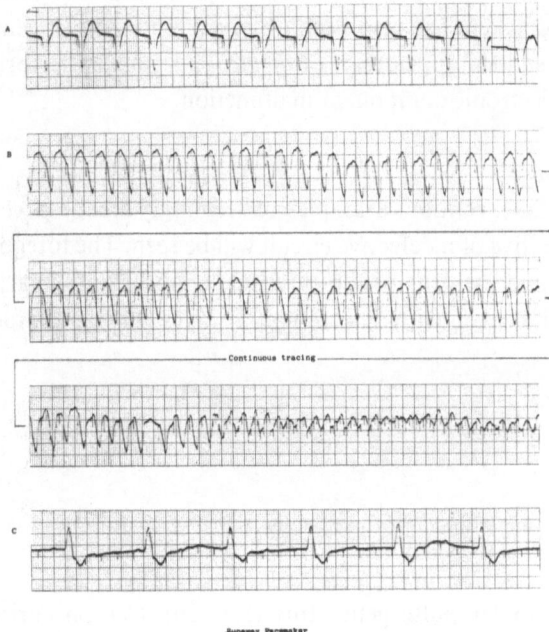

Figure 23. EKG rhythm strip showing pacemaker 'runaway' (Medtronic model 5860C). The lower strip shows the idioventricular escape rhythm after emergency interruption of the electrode.

and averages 0.1% per month. The incidence varies from one model to another and one soon comes to recognize 'good' models and 'bad' models. The usual manifestation of electronic circuit malfunction is the acute onset of a change in the expected performance of the system. This may vary from slight fluctuations in the basic stimulation rate, detectable only by digital counting through com-

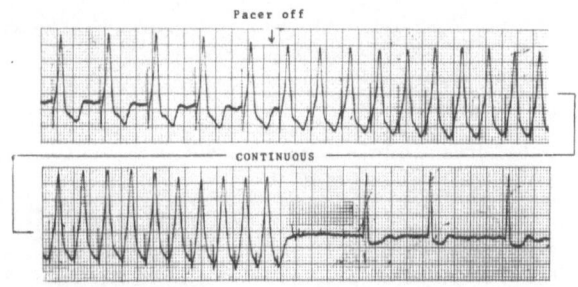

Figure 24. EKG rhythm strip showing pacemaker 'runaway' of a temporary (Electrodyne Model TR-3) pacemaker coincident with turning it off. Note the waning amplitude of the runaway stimulus with loss of capture as the output falls.

pletely chaotic pacemaker performance (Fig. 22), pacemaker runaway (Fig. 23) to sudden (and sometimes fatal) cessation of pacemaker function. Runaway of temporary pacemakers has also been observed (Fig. 24). In general, it can be stated that the sudden appearance of *illogical* pacemaker performance is commonly due to electronic component malfunction.

D. *Miscellaneous*

From time to time, random examples of seemingly erratic pacemaker performance not reflective of a defective circuit will be seen. The foregoing discussion has illustrated undersensing of sub-threshold endocardial signals. Occasionally oversensing will be seen with detection of T waves (Fig. 25) or local myopoten-

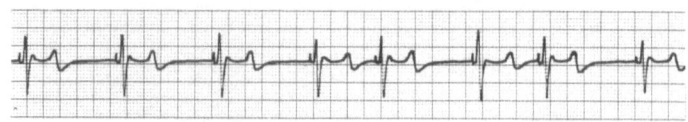

Figure 25. EKG rhythm strip showing 'oversensing' with sporadic recycling of pacemaker by the T wave (American Optical temporary pacemaker).

tials around unipolar pulse generators (Fig. 26). Certain curiosities may be identified at the time of pulse generator replacement which, if unrecognized, may simulate electronic malfunctions (Fig. 27-30).

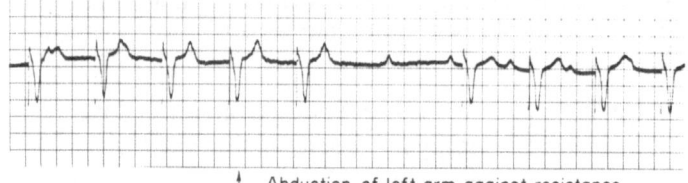

└─Abduction of left arm against resistance

Figure 26. EKG rhythm strip showing suppression of the pacemaker output during forceful abduction of left arm against resistance due to myopotential inhibition (unipolar pacemaker, Coratomic L-500 pulse generator in left pectoral area).

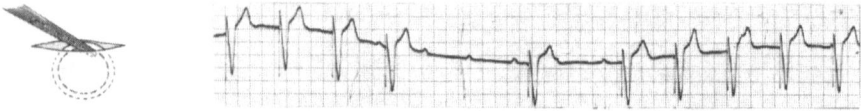

Figure 27. Effect of tapping metallic instrument against the indifferent lead of a unipolar ventricular inhibited generator (Cordis omnistanicor Model 162).

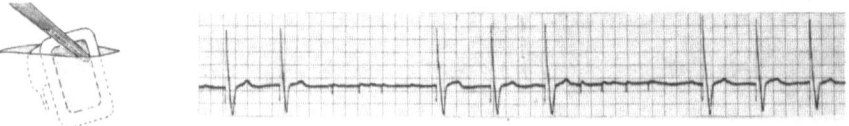

Figure 28. Effect of tapping metallic instrument against the indifferent lead of a unipolar ventricular tracking pacemaker (Starr Edwards Model 8114).

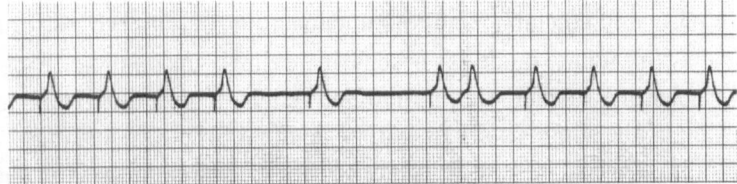

Figure 29. EKG rhythm strip showing electrostatic suppression of the output-stimulus caused by handling a silicone rubber coated pacemaker with dry rubber surgical gloves (Medtronic model 5842, 1974).

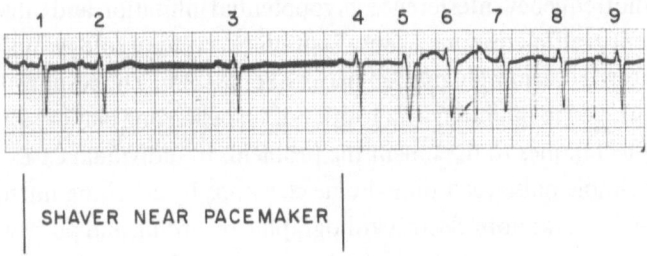

Figure 30. EKG rhythm strip showing external radiofrequency suppression of a temporary (atrial) pacemaker. (Medtronic model 5800 external pacer; Norelco shaver).

Conclusion

The foregoing review is intended to provide an overview of various types of malfunctions seen with temporary or permanent implantable pacemakers. A practical approach toward definition of the problem under study is encouraged. Before incriminating complex electronic malfunction it is appropriate to confirm stability and integrity of electrode connections and continuity through visual examination and careful review of overpenetrated chest x-rays. Manual manipulation of the pacemaker generator and attached lead and changes in body position may elicit failure due to loose connections or lead fracture. Abnormalities of sensing and or capture during the early period following implantation often herald perforation of the heart by the lead particularly when it remains within the cardiac silhouette on x-ray. Occasionally, faulty sensing reflects a low endocardial signal below the sensitivity of the sensing circuit of the pacemaker in use. It is useful to note that endocardial stimulation thresholds rise during the first 10 days following insertion – often by two or three fold while endocardial signal strength falls to return later to 80% of the control value. With marginal values at the time of initial implantation early evidence of erratic pacemaker performance may be seen during convalescence with later return to normal without necessarily requiring revision. Electronic circuit or component malfunction is typically characterized by unpredictable and often dangerous pacemaker performance. Fortunately this failure mode has become increasingly uncommon. Evidence of battery depletion with mercury zinc powered systems is most often characterized by slowing of the stimulation rate with widening of the stimulus pulse width. With lithium powered systems, evidence of battery depletion varies. A dual rate plateau is seen with Saft Lithium pacers while most of the remainder show a slow gradual decline in rate with an arbitrary end of life indicator averaging 6-8 pulses per minute. A variety of subtle anomalies of pacemaker performance induced by external radiofrequency interference, myopotential inhibition and intermittency of component malfunction may cause sporadic symptomatology in the patient with an otherwise seemingly normal pacemaker system. The responsible physician is encouraged to maintain a high index of suspicion and employ all available monitoring techniques to document the problem. In individual cases, this may range from simple pulse recording, home checkups by a visiting nurse or other home care service, random electrocardiographic recording and pulse wave form analysis to more sophisticated use of telemetric recordings and transtelephonic monitoring.

Literature

1. Birch, L.M., Berger, M. and Thomas, P.A., Synchronous diaphragmatic contraction: A complication of transvenous cardiac pacing. *Am. J. Cardiol.* 21, 88, 1968.
2. Blaser, R., Dittrich, H., Kirsch, U. und Schaldach, M., Electromagnetische Felder als Gefahrenquelle für Schrittmacherpatienten. *Dtsch. med. Wschr.* 97, 559, 1972.
3. Burchell, H.B., Hidden hazards of cardiac pacemakers (editorial). *Circulation* 24, 161, 1961.
4. Cosby, R.S., Poenido, J.R.F. and Cotton, B.H., Catheter perforation of the ventricle after intracardiac pacing. *Geriatrics* 22, 182, 1967.
5. Dekker, E., Buller, J. and Schuilenburg, R.M., Aids to electrical diagnosis for pacemaker failure. *Am. Heart J.* 70, 739, 1965.
6. Gerst, P.H., Bowman, F.O., Fleming, W.H. and Malm, J.R., Evaluation of pacemaker function and failure. *J. Thoracic, Cardiovascular Surg.* 54, 92, 1967.
7. Furman, S., Escher, D.J.W., Lister, J. and Schwedel, J.B., A comprehensive schema for management of pacemaker malfunction. *Ann. Surg.* 163, 611, 1966.
8. Furman, S. and Escher, D.J.W., Retained endocardial pacemaker electrodes. *J. Thoracic, Cardiovascular Surg.* 55, 737, 1968.
9. Furman, S. and Escher, D.J.W., *Principles and Techniques of Cardiac Pacing.* Harper and Row, New York 177-198, 1970.
10. Harthorne, J.W., Austen, W.G., Corning, H.C., McNamara, J.J. and Sanders, C.A., Technique and results of endocardial pacing in the elderly patient. *Circulation* 34, 124 (Suppl.) (abstract). Also, American Coll. of Phys. Regional Meeting, 1966, (Montreal), *Annals Int. Med.* 66, 831, 1967.
11. Harthorne, J.W., DeSanctis, R.W., Sulit, Y.Q.M., Sanders, C.A. and Austen, W.G., Epicardial versus endocardial pacemakers: Analysis of 109 cases. *Annals Thoracic Surg.* 6, 417, 1968.
12. Harthorne, J.W., Dinsmore, R.E. and DeSanctis, R.W., Superior vena caval anomaly preventing pervenous pacemaker implantation. *Brit Heart J.* 31, 809, 1969.
13. Harthorne, J.W., Preliminary Experience with The Starr-Edwards and Cordis Omnicor Pacemaker Systems. *Proceedings IVth International Symposium on Cardiac Pacing, Groningen 1973.* Royal Van Gorcum, Assen 349, 1974.

14. Kalmar, P., Bally, K.V., Kitzing, J., Krebber, H.J., Pinich, P. and Polonius, M.J., Clinical Complications due to Pacemaker System Failures and their management. *Advances in Pacemaker Technology*. Schaldach, M. and Furman, S., eds. Springer, Berlin 1975.

15. Kirsch, U., Kalmar, P., Rodewald, G. und Westermann, K.W., Spätkomplikationen der Herzschrittmachertherapie und ihre Behandlung. *Langenbecks Arch. Klin. Chir.* 329, 595, 1971.

16. Lillehei, C.W., Cruz, A.B., Johnsrude, I. and Sellers, R.D., A new method of assessing the state of charge of implanted cardiac pacemaker batteries. *Am. J. Cardiol.* 16, 17, 1965.

17. Lister, J.W., Furman, S., Stein, E., Damato, A.N., Schwedel, J.B. and Escher, D.J.W., A rapid determination of pacemaking defects in patients with artificial pacemakers. *Bull. N.Y. Acad. Med.* 40, 982, 1964.

18. Mymin, D., Cuddy, T.E., Sinha, S.N. and Winter, D.A., Inhibition of demand pacemakers by skeletal muscle potentials. *J. Am. Med. Ass.* 223, 527, 1973.

19. Noordjik, J.A., Oey, F.T.I. and Tebra, W., Myocardial electrodes and the danger of ventricular fibrillation. *Lancet* 1, 975, 1961.

20. Ormond, R.S., Rubenfire, M. and Anbe, D.T., Radiographic demonstration of myocardial penetration of permanent endocardial pacemakers. *Radiology* 98, 35, 1971.

21. Palmer, T.E., Finestone, A.J., Leary, J., Pacemaker induced diaphragmatic contractions. *J. Am. Med. Ass.* 200, 1179, 1967.

22. Parsonnet, V., Gilbert, L., Zucker, I.R. and Asa, M.M., Complications of the implanted pacemaker. A scheme for determining the cause of the defect and methods for correction. *J. Thoracic, Cardiovascular Surg.* 45, 801, 1963.

23. Parsonnet, V., Zucker, I.R., Kannerstein, M.L., Gilbert, L. and Alvares, J.F., The fate of permanent intracardiac electrodes. *J. Surg, Res.* 6, 285, 1966.

24. Peleska, B, and Buda, J., Stimulation of the phrenic nerve as a complication of implanted battery pacemaker: Management without thoracotomy. *J. Cardiac Surg.* 6, 477, 1965.

25. Richter, Arnauld, H.P., Thiem, E. und Westermann, K.W., Interferenzprobleme bei der Schrittmacherbehandlung. *Med. Klin.* 69, 1500, 1974.

26. Robboy, S.J., Harthorne, J.W., Leinbach, R.C., Sanders, C.A. and Austen, W.G., Autopsy findings with permanent pervenous pacemakers. *Circulation* 39, 495, 1969.

27. Rodewald, G., Giebel, O., Harms, H. und Scheppokat, K.D., Vorteile und Probleme der Anwendung vorhofgesteuerter Schrittmacher. *Langebecks Arch. Klin. Chir.* 313, 600, 1965.

28. Sowton, E. and Davies, J.G., Investigation of failure of artificial pacing. *Brit. Med. J.* 1, 1470, 1964.

29. Sowton, E., Detection of impending pacemaker failure. *Israel J. Med. Sci.* 3, 260, 1967.

30. Sprinkle, J.D., Takaro, T. and Scott, S.M., Phrenic nerve stimulation as a complication of the implantable cardiac pacemaker. *Circulation* 28, 114, 1963.

31. Whalen, R.E., Starmer, F. and McIntosh, H.D., Electrical hazards associated with cardiac pacing. *Ann. N.Y. Acad. Sci.* 111, 922, 1964.

32. Wirtzfeld, A., Lampadius, M. und Ruprecht, E.O., Unterdrückung von Demand-Schrittmachern durch Muskelpotentiale. *Dtsch. med. Wschr.* 97, 61, 1972.

AN APPRAISAL OF PACEMAKER FOLLOWUP TECHNIQUES

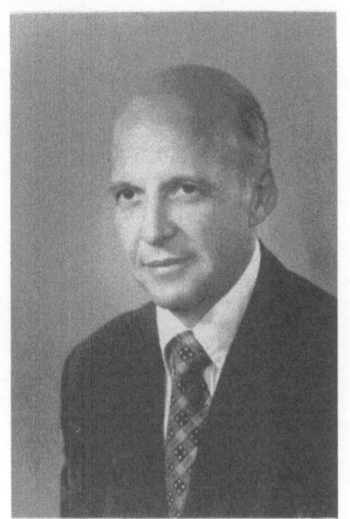

Dr. Victor Parsonnet received his undergraduate training at Cornell University (1945), medical degree at New York University (1947) and interned in surgery at the Beth Israel hospital in Boston, Massachusetts. Two years of residency in Pathology and five further years of surgical residency were followed by a cardiovascular surgical fellowship with Dr. Michael DeBakey in Houston, Texas. He is currently Director of Surgery at the Newark Beth Israel Hospital, Newark, New Jersey, and Clinical Professor of Surgery at the New Jersey College of Medicine and Dentistry, Newark, New Jersey. He is a member of many national and international medical societies and well known in the field of cardiac pacing for his many contributions to the advancement of pacemaker technology.

AN APPRAISAL OF PACEMAKER FOLLOWUP TECHNIQUES *

VICTOR PARSONNET, M.D., GEORGE MYERS, PH.D., MARJORIE MANHARDT,
LAWRENCE GILBERT, M.D. AND I. RICHARD ZUCKER, M.D.

with the technical assistance of Esther Shilling and Ann Marie Elliff

Where as a 1972 survey revealed that only half the pacemaker centers in the United States had organized follow-up systems for their patients, a survey in 1975 indicates a growing conviction that a follow-up system is essential for patient care, and in fact such a service is provided by about 90% of the physicians (1, 2). It is evident that most patients with implanted pacemakers in the United States are now followed in some fashion. Approximately 68% of centers use telephone monitoring, 71% have pacemaker 'clinics' most in conjunction with telephone analysis, and only 8% have no follow-up system at all.

Follow-up techniques vary greatly, particularly with regard to devices, schedules, physical setting, degree of patient-physician contact, administration, and institutional or private affiliation. Every pacemaker surveillance system is based upon the observation that the characteristics of the electrical output of a pulse generator are affected by the battery voltage. The manufacturers eventually designed their pacemakers to slow down as battery voltage dropped, and today, no matter what battery is used, there will be a drop in output voltage and rate in almost all instances of battery failure.

Analysis of the electrical output of the pacemaker will also detect other changes in pulse generator characteristics, such as rate, impulse amplitude, duration, shape, and area (3). It is also possible to assess the integrity of the pulse generator sensing circuit and its refractory period (4).

Methods of pacemaker output evaluation

There are various ways in which the output parameters of the pacemaker may be studied. The pulse generator rate (or interval) measured directly or indirectly over the telephone, may be evaluated in its free running (automatic) rate, and in its magnet rate (disabling the sensing circuit); in some cases it is necessary to

* From the Department of Surgery and the Pacemaker Center of the Newark Beth Israel Medical Center and the New Jersey Medical School, Newark, N.J.
Supported in part by grant # 3 IG03RM0042-01 of the New Jersey Regional Medical Program, and by the Pacemaker Foundation.

evaluate the differences between these two rates. The interval is measured best with a digital counter, or directly by computer. Taking the pulse manually is feasible but less accurate and more time consuming (5).

The output impulse duration is usually taken from a photograph of the output waveform, by measurement of the elapsed time between the leading and trailing edges of the pulse. It may also be done on a digital counter or with a home device that converts the interval to an audio signal for telephone transmission. Measuring the pulse duration is becoming more important because some pulse generators are designed to show a change in pulse duration with a drop in battery voltage, while others that are programmable may show changes in this parameter at different programmed rates.

Impulse amplitude is a difficult parameter to measure precisely because it varies with respiration and body position. Therefore the patient must be studied in an identical position each time. The output may be measured directly from a photograph of the waveform or by computer. The impulse shape also may be analyzed by inspection of the waveform photograph. Although one phone device is capable of measuring the output area and another the output amplitude, these devices are not in wide general use.

The sensing circuit and pulse generator refractory period are evaluated in different ways. When spontaneous cardiac contractions occur normal function of the sensing circuit will be obvious because appropriate triggering or inhibition of the pulse generator will be seen on the electrocardiogram. But when the heart is captured continually by the pacemaker it may be necessary to use external overdrive (application of a second pacemaker impulse to the chest wall over the implanted pulse generator) to test the sensing circuit (4). Changing the rate of the external impulse will allow the observer to estimate the refractory period. This will be the difference between the interval of the latest impulse after the R wave that fails to inhibit the pacemaker, and the first impulse to inhibit it. Rapid external overdrive will 'turn off' the implanted pulse generator and thereby will permit evaluation of the underlying unpaced electrocardiogram. (With bipolar pacemakers this test is often more difficult or impossible, because the amplitude of the external overdrive pulse as 'seen' by the electrodes in the heart is too small.)

In addition to evaluating the output of the pulse generator, follow-up care includes interviewing, examining, and counseling the patient. Whether or not this service should be provided in the private physician's office or in a pacemaker clinic depends upon the available setting and on individual preference. Most clinics are hospital based, but many are held in a private office, and others are being conducted by proprietary services. (A list of these is provided in the appendix.)

Of the many methods of follow-up, the most popular is the pacemaker clinic that combines waveform analysis and transtelephone monitoring; the next most popular is transtelephone monitoring alone.

There is no general agreement on the best method, for the 'best' is obviously determined by the patient load, the patient's distance from the center, and whether the patient is well enough to travel. To compare and evaluate all of the possible variations of the methods of follow-up is difficult, but it is probably fair to say that the more thorough the examination and the more carefully it is performed the more accurate will be the detection of pacemaker problems.

One basic issue is the evaluation of the relative merits of the two most commonly used followup systems – transtelephone monitoring alone, and clinic waveform analysis plus transtelephone monitoring. We have described our clinic at the Newark Beth Israel Medical Center in detail in previous reports, and since then there have been only a few changes. The number of affiliated centers has increased to 10, with centers distributed throughout the state. Each center uses the same system, and the same computer, a DEC PDP-11. At the Newark Beth Israel Medical Center, where innovations are tested first, the waveform oscilloscope has been replaced by the Gutmann apparatus. In order to speed up clinic procedures and minimize errors, a pacemaker analyzer, manufactured by L.P.G. Gutmann, has been used in conjunction with a Hewlett-Packard thermal printer to measure waveform data and automatically record them. The analyzer, when connected to the patient with three electrocardiographic leads, automatically measures the pulse interval, pulse amplitude, and pulse width of the artifact from the implanted pacemaker and displays these quantities digitally. (The time constant of the pulse decay is also measured, but is not used in our clinic.) The pulse waveform shape is also displayed on a cathode ray tube for photography. The digital values are used to operate the printer, thus permitting a recording of all data without the necessity of having an operator write anything down, a step which is both time consuming and error prone.

The pacemaker analyzer, in its standard form, will not measure artifact parameters unless the pulse amplitude, as measured at the skin, is greater than approximately 40 mv. Modifications made by the manufacturer at the request of the Pacemaker Center increased the analyzer's sensitivity so that artifacts as small as 6 mv may be measured. Thus, parameters for all units, except for a few using bipolar electrodes, may be determined rapidly and accurately.

y   The chief problem with a clinic system as described is that it requires substantial organization and administration. Moreover, it is not always convenient, and at times it is impossible for patients to travel to the clinic. In these instances greater reliance is placed on transtelephone monitoring. Incidentally, because the two methods differ in frequency of checkup, the overall costs to the patient are not increased by a clinic.

Transtelephone monitoring is relatively simple, but it provides limited information. A monitor has two basic functions, namely transmitting an electrocardiogram, and providing an accurate digital readout of the impulse interval. All of the devices now offered do this. But the transmitters of one manufacturer cannot, in general, be used with the receivers of another manufacturer because the method of detecting the artifact differs from unit to unit. The pacemaker artifact cannot be sent directly over the telephone lines – its location must be indicated by some type of 'code,' and the different manufacturers have selected different codes. While sometimes the electrocardiogram may be picked up on a receiver of a different manufacturer than the transmitter, usually the pulse interval measurement circuitry will not work. (A consequence of these 'codes' is that the received artifact often has the wrong polarity.)

Recently a number of new pacemaker telephone monitors have been offered for sale. Physically, some are quite small and light. The methods for attaching electrodes differ, with some units having electrodes that are somewhat difficult for elderly people to attach. Some units have the facility for the data taker to signal the patient. Central receiving units differ considerably in size, ease of use, and cost. Some require an adjustment by the operator to receive accurate rates and electrocardiograms, while others are virtually automatic. A new unit, just recently announced, also measures pulse width over the telephone.

Despite these considerable improvements in equipment, technical artifacts of various types continue to appear. These electrocardiographic distortions are often confusing, and almost always require a visit to the clinic for more careful analysis of the problem.

Finally, telephone monitoring alone fails to provide the doctor-patient contact that is a basic ingredient of satisfactory care.

Problems faced in follow-up care.
Proliferation of information and patient population

The 1975 survey revealed that there were approximately 156,000 people living with pacemakers in the United States or one in 1,300 of the population. (The total number must now be closer to 200,000.) Thus, any pacemaker center is likely to have many patients with many clinical conditions, with varied and unusual indications for pacing, and often with complex rhythm disturbances. There will also be a great variety of pulse generators and models. Even if one chooses to use the models of just one company, there will always be new models by that company. Often it is necessary to study patients from other centers where different types of pacemakers are being used. To illustrate, in 1975 we used the pacemakers listed in Table 1, but we are presently following patients with 49 different model pulse generators from 13 companies. Just to keep track of this

MFG.	AS Iˢᵗ IMPLANT	AS REPLACEMENT	TOTAL
CORDIS	35	66	101
MEDTRONIC	18	15	33
CPI	19	10	29
ARCO	10	8	18
ESB-MEDCOR	1	2	3
INTERMEDICS	3	–	3
STARR-EDWARDS	–	2	2
GE	1	1	2
BIOTRONIK	1	–	1
A.O. BIFOCAL	1	–	1
NUCLEARS ARCO	6	10	16
CORATOMIC	3	6	9
MEDTRONIC	4	3	7
CORDIS	3	1	4
TOTALS	105	124 (54%)	229

Table 1. New pulse generators implanted. 1975 (12-31-75).

Table 2. Pacer data for hot line.

Manufacturer and model
100% warranty time
Manufacturer's recommended removal date
Pacing mode
Power source and number of cells
Output characteristics (e.g. pulse duration, automatic rate, magnetic rate, output, etc)
Special features
Predicted and known failure modes

---

amount of information, we have established a 'hot line' that contains the information shown in Table 2. This makes it possible for us, as well as for the centers affiliated with us, to acquire instant information with regard to failure modes and other problems that might arise in the course of patient care.

New devices

New pulse generators are developed all the time. The most important innovation has been the utilization of new power sources. Eight different lithium pacemakers by American companies are now on the market, each with different failure modes.» The *predicted* decay modes of these batteries are shown in figure

* List of companies: ARCO, Coratomic, Cordis, CPI, Intermedics, Medcor, Medtronic, Starr-Edwards.

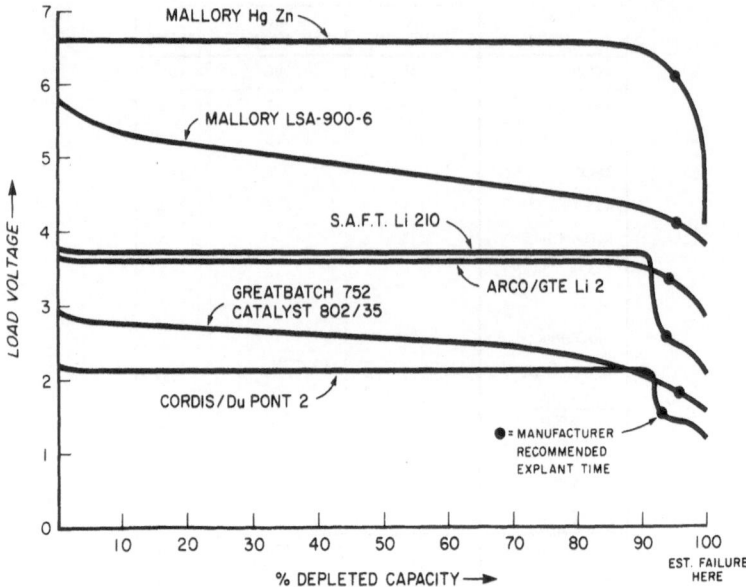

Figure 1. Diagrammatic representations of drop in battery voltage of various types of lithium batteries as compared to a classical mercury-zinc cell (top).

1. Experience tells us that these estimates must not be accepted at face value, and that only observation and time will tell what the real situation will be. A study of the first Greatbatch (CPI) cell, for example, in which it was predicted that after 3 years there would be a 2-4 beat change in the rate as the interval impedance of the battery built up has, in 15 units, so far shown no change in rate at all after an average of 34.5 months (range 30-43 months). (There were minor changes within a range of + 10 to − 9 milliseconds.) It is not clear whether this means that battery performance is better than anticipated, or that concomitant changes in

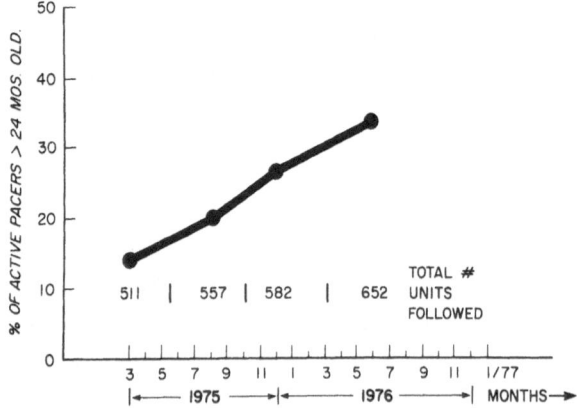

Figure 2. Increase in percentage of patients with pacemakers over 24 months old.

function of some of the components counter-balanced the early drop in battery output. But the observed findings are clearly different than anticipated, and therefore one cannot predict *with confidence* what will happen next.

The use of long life batteries has begun to have a tangible impact on the age of the implanted pacemakers. In our clinic the percentage of patients whose pacers are more than 24 months old has increased from 15% to 32% in one year (Figure 2).

There has also been an increase in the age of the pulse generators removed for battery exhaustion (Figure 3), after there seemed to be a plateau of 21-22 months

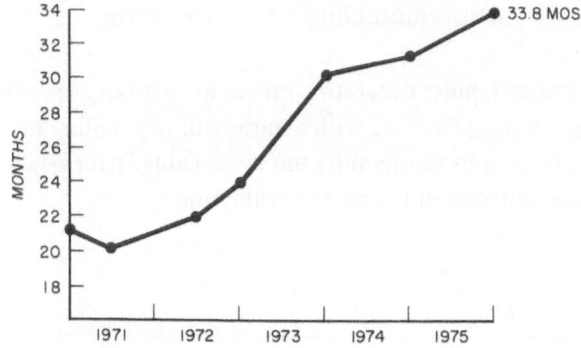

Figure 3. Increase in average pulse generator age removed for documented battery exhaustion.

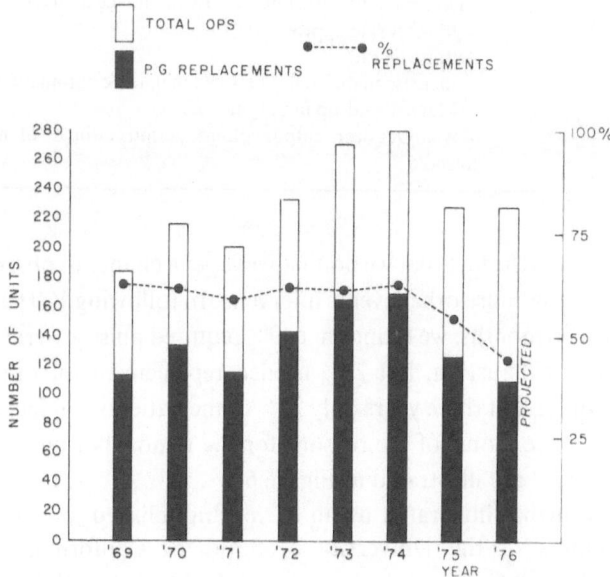

Figure 4. Ratio of operations for pulse generator replacement to all pacemaker operations by years 1976 figure is extrapolated from data of the first 6 months of the year.

for several years. In 1972 this began to change so that in 1975 the average age of pulse generators removed for battery exhaustion was almost 34 months. Likewise, the ratio of operations for pulse generator replacement to total operations has begun to fall, after it was 59% to 62% for several years (Figure 4).

These facts, albeit happy ones, increase the burden of pacemaker surveillance by increasing the time that the pacemakers must be followed, and making us less certain about the eventual manifestations that represent inevitable signs of battery exhaustion.

Unpredictability of failure modes

As already mentioned, pulse generators do not always fail as predicted. To add to the problem, we are presented with a variety of new failure modes designed into the pulse generator by the manufacturer (see Table 3); these new modes must be identified and understood for proper evaluation.

Table 3. Special EOL behavior.

	Sign
Medtronic & Cordis	Some of each – increase pulse width
Medcor 3-70B	– 2 Cell ↓ in one stack → Increased automatic rate, & 7 BPM change in magnet rate
ARCO Nuclear VVI	– Magnet rate approaches Automatic rate
AO Predicta	– Increase in difference between magnet & automatic rate
Elema 169C	– Magnet → drop in output
Vitatron Optimel	– Analyzer decr. output voltage, permits estimate of impedance and treshold

Important, too, is the fact that we don't always get a chance to observe end-of-life battery failure because other events intervene. In following 100 patients who lived for at least 36 months, we found that 49% required pulse generator replacement for battery exhaustion, but 29% needed replacement for other reasons (Figure 5). At the end of three years only 22% of the patients still had their pulse generators in service. Some of the reasons for the removal of pulse generators over a 5 year period are illustrated in Figure 6.

This issue is further illustrated by an as yet unpublished joint study of the pacemaker centers of the University of Southern California, Montefiore Hospital and Medical Center in the Bronx, and the Newark Beth Israel Medical Center (6). A preliminary report of the first two years shows that only 47% of pulse generators were removed for battery exhaustion, and the remainder for a

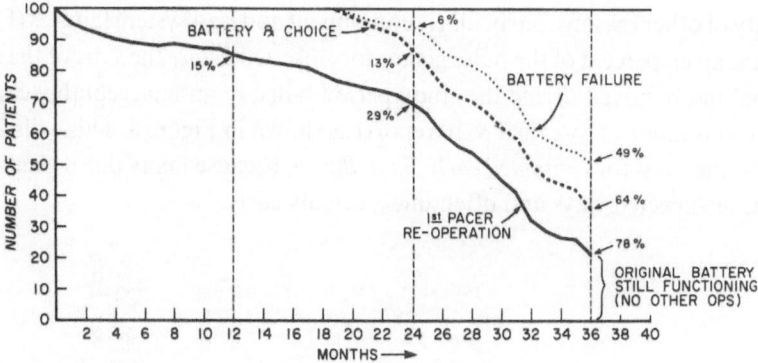

Figure 5. Reoperation of pulse generator replacement in 100 consecutive patients followed at least 36 months (see text).

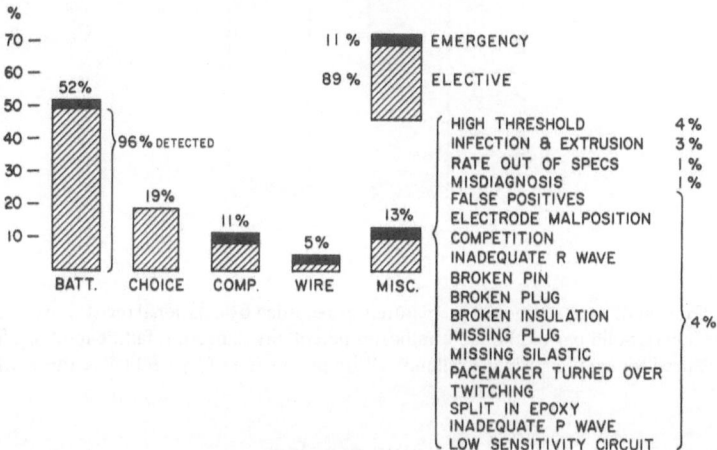

Figure 6. Reasons for pulse generator replacement at the Newark Beth Israel Medical Center over a 5 year period (1971-1975). All causes – 669 cases.

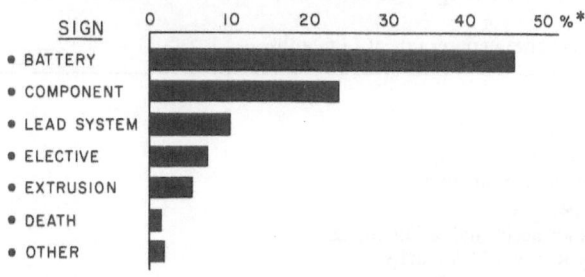

Figure 7. Documented reasons for pulse generator replacement from a joint registry program over a two-year period (with permission of Drs. Bilitch & Furman). All units – 773 (of 2118). (6).

variety of other reasons, particularly component and lead system failures (Figure 7). Seventeen percent of the pulse generators inserted *before* the start of the study period and removed *during* the study period failed in an unacceptably early or dangerous mode (a so-called & 10 report) as shown in Figure 8. This calls attention to the need for *continued early surveillance*, because many pulse generators fail in unexpected ways and often unexpectedly early.

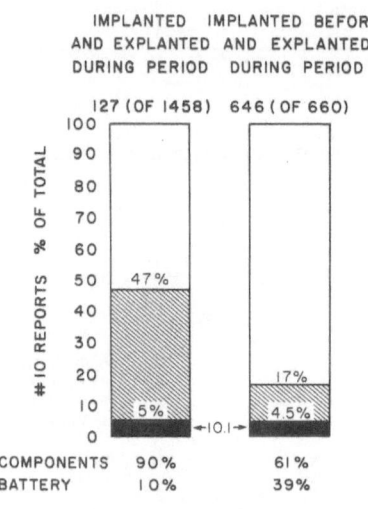

Figure 8. Percent of pacers removed prematurely as recorded by a national registry over a two-year period (see text). Solid bar of about 5% indicates potentially dangerous failure modes. These data emphasize need for careful *early* surveillance. (With permission of Drs. Bilitch & Furman). (6).

Sample problem

To emphasize the need for a thorough evaluation system of implanted pulse generators, it may be helpful to look at a relatively simple, but rather frequent

Table 4. Sudden change in pacer rate at 14 months.

Possible causes –
   Abnormal drop in battery voltage
   Normal drop in battery voltage
   Change in component function
   Change in impedance
   Reprogramming, accidental or intentional
   Triggering by R wave in VVT units
   EMI (including myopotential)
   Partial recycling by potential other than R wave (after potentials, T waves)
   Cardiac arrhythmias inhibiting pacer
   Broken wire or connector – make & break

---

problem that one might see in the clinic. Table 4 shows the diagnostic possibilities when a pulse generator rate change is found 14 months after implantation. To solve this diagnostic puzzle one must know the various ways of evaluating a pulse generator and, more importantly, one must have *the facilities* to perform the needed tests, such as those shown in Table 5. Only an approach such as this will elucidate this specific difficulty, while phone transmission alone may not.

Table 5. Questions and actions

What kind of pacer? Programmable?
Any special failure modes?
Any injury, fall, unusual activity by patient?
Chest X-ray O.K.? Wire intact? Position unchanged?
Waveform normal?
Response to magnet?
Response to EOD?
Study ECG for sources of recycling?
Any special tests to be done?

Discussion

The great variety of problems serves to emphasize the need for frequent follow-up evaluations. There has been no generally accepted schedule, although certain generalizations may be made. Because there are so many pacemaker failures related to factors *other than* battery exhaustion, because of the complexity of clinical situations, and because of the growing numbers of patients, clinical indications, devices, special detection devices, and failure modes, fairly frequent follow-up must be continued *throughout the life* of the pulse generator. This is best accomplished by combining transtelephonic monitoring with periodic clinic

Table 6. Advantages of a waveform clinic plus telephone monitoring.

1. Direct patient contact
interviews
examination
instruction
reassurance
2. Accuracy of diagnosis
detailed ECG (or other)
chest X-ray
external overdrive
3. Direct intervention
reprogramming
4. Extension of pacer life

visits that include waveform analysis and other ancillary procedures. The frequency of tests should be modified when a problem is suspected. Pacemaker follow-up by telephone alone is inadequate because it does not provide all the parameters seen in Table 6.

Based on a previous examination of our own data we have estimated that the full analysis will extend pacer life by 15% over phone (rate) analysis alone. Moreover, the age of pacers removed for battery failure on the basis of a telephone proprietary service (Cardiac Datacorp) reveals that with this method the average age of explanted pulse generators is 27 months, while at the Newark Beth Israel Medical Center the average age is 35.5 months, an increase of 31% (8).

Conclusion

Pacemaker followup will continue to grow more complex, not less so, as heretofore anticipated. Therefore, a sound surveillance system must be established. The method should combine waveform analysis in the clinic and regular transtelephonic monitoring.

Literature

1. Parsonnet, V., A survey of cardiac pacing in the United States and Canada. Proceedings IVth International Symposium on *Cardiac Pacing, Groningen 1973.* Royal Van Gorcum, Assen 41-48, 1974.
2. Parsonnet, V., Survey of pacing in the U.S.A., 1975. *Proceedings Vth International Symposium on Cardiac Pacing, Tokyo 1976.* Editor, Y. Watanabe. Excerpta Medica, Amsterdam 1977.
3. Parsonnet, V., Myers, G.H., Gilbert, L., Zucker, I.R. and Shilling, E., Follow-up of implanted pacemakers. *Amer. Heart. J.* 87, 642-653, 1974.
4. Parsonnet, V., Myers, G.H., Gilbert, L., Zucker, I.R. and Rockland, R., A regional network of clinics for analysis of implanted pacemakers. *Cardiac Arrhythmias*, Dreifus, Leonard, S. and Likoff, William Eds. Grune & Stratton, New York 1973.
5. Gordon, A.F., Pacemaker follow-up with transistor radio and stopwatch. *Chest* 66, 557, 1974.
6. Bilitch, M., Furman, S. and Parsonnet, V., Unpublished data from a joint registry.
7. Parsonnet, V., et al: Follow-up of implanted pacemakers: an evaluation of surveillance methods. *Diagnostic Methods in Cardiology. Fowler, Anne O., Ed., F.A. Davis, Philadelphia 431-446, 1975.*
8. Stern, T., *Cardiac Datacorp. Personal communication.*

AVAILABLE PHONE DEVICES

	FUNCTION OF EQUIPMENT
ESB, INC. 5920 RODMAN ST. HOLLYWOOD, FLA.	INTERVAL, ECG & PULSE WIDTH
INSTROMEDIX, INC. GREENTREE BUSINESS PARK 10950 S.W. FIFTH BEAVERTON, OREGON 97005	INTERVAL & ECG
COMPUTER INSTRUMENTS CORP. 92 MADISON AVE. HEMPSTEAD, L.I., N.Y. 11550	INTERVAL & ECG
MEDTRONIC, INC. TELETRACE 3055 OLD HIGHWAY EIGHT MINNEAPOLIS, MINN. 55418	INTERVAL & ECG
CORDIS CORP. 125 NORTHEAST 40TH ST. MIAMI, FLA. 33137	INTERVAL & ECG
SURVIVAL TECHNOLOGY, INC. CARDIO-BEEPER 7811 WOODMONT AVE. BETHESDA, MD. 20014	INTERVAL & ECG
CENTERLINE, INC. 7425 S.W. 42ND ST. MIAMI, FLA. 33155	INTERVAL & ECG
ARCO MEDICAL PRODUCTS CO. P.O. BOX 546 LEECHBURG, PA. 15656	INTERVAL & ECG
PIONEER MEDICAL SYSTEMS AQUONICS, INC. 10 ROCKDALE ST. WORCESTER, MASS. 01606	INTERVAL & ECG

PROPRIETARY PHONE SERVICES

CARDIAC DATACORP, INC. 1705 WALNUT ST. PHILADELPHIA, PA.	INTERVAL AND PERIPHERAL PULSE
PACEMAKER DIAGNOSTIC CLINIC OF AMERICA 4020 WEST NEWBERRY RD. GAINESVILLE, FLA. 32607	INTERVAL, AMPLITUDE, PULSE DURATION AND ECG
MEDALERT CORPORATION 301 E. 87TH ST. NEW YORK, N.Y. 10028	INTERVAL AND ECG
CARDIO-PACE EVALUATION, INC. 9999 S.W. WILSHIRE PORTLAND, OREGON 97225	INTERVAL AND ECG
CARDIOLABS INC. P.O. BOX 1794 DUXBURY, MASS. 02332	INTERVAL AND ECG

DEVICES SUPPLIED WITH PACER

EDWARDS PACEMAKER SYSTEMS DIV. OF AMER. HOSP. SUPPLY CO. 1923 S.E. MAIN ST. IRVINE, CALIFORNIA 92713	INTERVAL & ECG
GENERAL ELECTRIC CO. MEDICAL SYSTEMS DIVISION 4855 ELECTRIC AVENUE MILWAUKEE, WISCONSIN 53201	INTERVAL ONLY (ONLY FOR GE PACEMAKERS)

ROUND TABLE DISCUSSION

QUESTION

John Bete, M.D. (Cape Cod Hospital, Hyannis, Mass.): Does increasing the rate in a ventricular demand pacemaker chronically implanted increase cardiac output in a patient with borderline ventricular failure? That is, is borderline ventricular failure an indication for implanting a rate adjustable pacemaker?

RESPONSE

J. Warren Harthorne, M.D.: I would have to respond by saying I honestly don't know because there are very few long term physiologic studies of the effect on cardiac output by increased rate of cardiac stimulation. The information that is available comes from Dr. Furman and Escher, Dr. Samet, Dr. Parsonnet, and others which would suggest that there is an inverse relationship between the augmentation of cardiac output by a rising stimulation rate and the integrity of myocardial contractility. A person with an abnormal heart damaged by cardio-myopathy, ischemic heart disease or fibrosis is less able to respond to the increasing rate and frequently drops the stroke volume as the rate rises and ends up with approximately the same cardiac output in contrast to the younger individual with a well preserved myocardium where increase in the heart rate may result in an increased cardiac output. Some disturbing studies would suggest that the early increase in cardiac output obtained with a faster rate of stimulation is not sustained. If you take those patients back into the laboratory twenty-four hours later, you'll find that with the slightly increased rate of stimulation, their cardiac output will be back where it was when you started. We badly need some type of noninvasive technique for recording the cardiac output in these patients with atrial pacing, AV sequential pacing and programmable ventricular stimulators so we can actually add credibility to our suspicions.

QUESTION

Paul A. Levine, M.D., (University Hospital, Boston, Mass.): Is a 'prophylactic demand pacemaker' indicated in a patient who has survived an acute anterior wall infarction during which complete heart block developed but following which sinus rhythm was restored. This particular patient not only developed heart block during the acute infarction which required a temporary pacemaker, but then reverted to sinus.

Thomas Preston, M.D.: As a general rule, I would. There have been several papers and reports published on this subject. Initially I believe it was Atkins and his group who reported a series of six patients whom they have accumulated over several years who had had this phenomenon of transient complete heart block with return to conducted rhythm during infarction and then who had sudden death. From that time on, they examined their patients more carefully and implanted permanent pacemakers in everyone who had transient complete heart block. The survival of this group of 12 or 14 patients wasn't much greater. It wasn't as long as one might hope for, presumably because these patients had big infarcts. There has been at least one conflicting report in this respect. It is still controversial, but my conclusion is that I think we should pace these patients. They are at high risk for sudden death. Atkins' statistics aren't perfect in that he doesn't have a randomized study. He did a retrospective study on patients who had a high degree of sudden death and then a prospective study in which he used only one type of treatment, that is pacing. Nevertheless, I would suspect that 10 or 20 percent of such patients can avoid sudden death by pacing. It may be much greater than that. We may only prolong life in these patients for six or seven months, but I would pace such people and do.

J. Warren Harthorne, M.D.: Excuse me Tom. There are a number of questions pertinent to this. I won't read them all, but there is also a question from Dr. Farag from Los Angeles pertaining to the indications for a right ventricular temporary electrode in a patient with left bundle branch block during cardiac catheterization. As a longstanding catheterizer, I absolutely would insert a temporary pacemaker electrode in the venous bed. I would not necessarily pass it into the right ventricle, but in the presence of documented instability of the conductive mechanism or in a patient with an anterior wall infarct with demonstrated complete heart block, the procedure of implanting a permanent transvenous pacemaker is relatively innocuous, and we would proceed without hesitation.

Thomas Preston, M.D.: Quick comment – watch out because you have probably seen the situation whereby passing a temporary pacer you produce right bundle branch block by putting it in the right ventricle and in the presence of prior left bundle branch block you produce complete heart block.

J. Warren Harthorne, M.D.: That's exactly why we don't put it in the ventricle.

We put it in the superior vena cava. We use a Zucker electrode which allows us not only to pace but to infuse fluids.

QUESTION

Paul M. Zoll, M.D.: Does anyone know of long term studies demonstrating significant reduction of cardiac output with AV dissociation which is not related to the rate? Does the simple loss of atrial transport, in and of itself, reduce cardiac output? Is the fall in cardiac output consequent to loss of atrial transport an acute event or is the effect sustained?

RESPONSE

Victor Parsonnet, M.D.: I just have an indirect answer that we don't really know much about cardiac output after the pacemaker is implanted until we develop some good noninvasive way of doing it. The classical paper by Adolph about five years ago was very interesting and very challenging and it has been bothering me for a long time. He studied a number of patients, somewhat less than 10, with cardiac output at a time of pulse generator implantation. The first determination measured the cardiac output before the pulse generator was turned on and after it was turned on and found a significant increase in cardiac output. Two years later when the patient returned for generator replacement, the cardiac output had fallen to where it was before the patient had a ventricular paced rhythm. There is something peculiar about cardiac output studies and perhaps peculiar about these patients.

Hilbert J. Th. Thalen, M.D.: I can add a little more to that comment. Some studies have been done in this respect in Cambridge by Edgar Sowton. He divided the patients into two groups; the first group clearly had congestive heart disease and the second group with heart block without signs of congestive heart disease, and the second group responded very well, but the other group did not. I know from my own experience from the clinic with a lot of patients with pacemakers that you do not cure the disease. A lot of these patients need digitalis and diuretics. We are now trying in some of these patients to implant atrial triggered units. So far, it has been very difficult for us to demonstrate really what an atrial contribution does do when you try to measure it. However, patients feel better, and I think this is because they can increase their cardiac output when they have to respond to sudden exercise; the first response is the frequency. On the long run, some of these patients with standard ventricular pacers go into congestive heart failure. About 20-25 percent of the deaths in patients with pacemakers are due to kidney failure or intractable heart failure. You see this after pacing for a long time and probably reflects a decrease in the cardiac output. We might be able, with atrial pacing, to improve that a little bit, but when patients reach that stage, they have a very high death incidence.

QUESTION

Maximiliaan Kaulbach, M.D. (Salem Hospital, Salem Mass.): What has happened to the biogalvanic pacing question? Can the problems of tissue overgrowth be overcome? Is there a real future for this self-perpetuating pacemaker? How does the biogalvanic pacemaker function?

RESPONSE

Josef K. Cywinski, Ph.D.: Well, I wish I knew a straight forward answer. I am biased. I put too much work into the biogalvanic pacemaker to say objectively there is no future. I think there is a future. I think the biogalvanic pacemaker may be competitive and may be a tentative choice to longstanding pacemakers. The tissue growth mechanism can be overcome, and we have clinical evidence to support the technological issues that are still surmounting, and we are working on it. It is only a matter of enough funds to continue that study. The basic principle of the biogalvanic system is a simple cathodic reaction which reduces oxygen on a catalytic platinum surface and by the way of reduction produces a flow of electrons in a connecting circuit. It is a fuel cell with a hybrid cathode. As an anode, to create an electrostatic field to drive these electrons and ions into conduction, a dissimilar metal has to be used. In the case of my device, it's zinc or in the case of the other investigators, zinc aluminum magnesium alloys. This zinc vs. platinum creates an electromotive force and actually the mechanism of production of oxygen drives the electrical carriers through the wires with this electromotive force. The disadvantage of a biogalvanic pacemaker is low voltage; they cannot and/or should not be stacked in series as other investigators in England have tried to do by putting interconnecting membranes in between. Whenever you put a membrane in a living system, you are asking for trouble or clogging of this membrane. I elected a clean open system without the membrane. The only thing I have had to deal with was the natural tissue membrane surrounding the biogalvanic cell, and the oxygen diffusion limitation via this surrounding tissue capsule. By proper choice of highly efficient materials like catalyst platinum compound similar to that used in catalytic converters for automobiles in the United States, one can work in a very low oxygen concentration environment and still produce enough electricity. There is not too much power required by contemporary pacemakers and pacemaker circuits.

QUESTION

Howard Corning, M.D. (Falmouth Hospital, Falmouth, Mass.): What is the significance of the low voltage of the lithium cell? Can they not be stacked?

RESPONSE

Josef K. Cywinski, Ph.D.: In some manufacturers' models, they are stacked.

However, the geometry of the connection of lithium cells in series poses a problem because they are large and they take up a lot of space and weight. Saft lithium cells are usually stacked because they are the smallest, a button size, but they don't have as large a capacity and expected longevity as others, such as Wilson Greatbatch or Catalyst Research lithium cells.

QUESTION

A. Azulay, M.D. (Central General Hospital, Plainview, NY): What are the advantages of coronary sinus electrodes over J-shaped atrial appendage leads?

RESPONSE

John Messenger, M.D.: My only comment would be that the J-shaped wires which we tried to implant several years ago were much more difficult to maintain in proper position. We have not used the wire spring type electrodes in the atrium except on rare occasions because we were concerned about tears in the atrial tissue. Sensing of the QRS seems to work well in the coronary sinus and it is reasonably simple to do. It's a method which we have been able to do readily day in and day out. I think the answers will not be in on that until a series of J-electrodes have been placed comparing the two in more patients.

J. Warren Harthorne, M.D.: I would just like to interject an editorial comment. We have had experience with about 60 atrial pacemakers using predominantly the coronary sinus lead demonstrated by Dr. Messinger and to a lesser extent the curved J-loop electrode. To date there has not been an ideal atrial pacing electrode available and one must maintain an inventory of different pieces of equipment. We have also used the American Optical J-loop lead. It is very difficult to explain verbally without illustrations the problems which one gets into with sensing by a demand pulse generator attached to an atrial lead. The demand pulse generator attached to a coronary sinus electrode will very often sense the QRS complex of its own stimulated beat, even though it is an atrial paced beat. In the presence of first degree block, the QRS comes alone, falls outside the refractory period of the pacemaker and recycles it. The alternative is to use a fixed rate pacemaker which is what we almost invariably use, a programmable fixed rate pacer on a coronary sinus lead. However, if you occasionally pace the ventricle via the coronary sinus electrode as the electrode slides back and forth in the coronary sinus, then you cannot use a fixed rate stimulator because you may precipitate a ventricular arrhythmia. In that setting a J-loop electrode in the atrial appendage may be desirable. So I think each electrode has its own role. We keep a variety in stock and we try one. If it doesn't work, we try another. You must record the amplitude of the complex coming back via the electrode as well as the stimulation amplitude. Excuse me for interrupting.

John Messenger, M.D.: Dr. John. Udall, who is on our staff and is Associate Professor at University of California at Irvine, placed his first atrial electrode in the atrial septum via a Brockenbrau catheter by using a technique which he has developed in animals and had an acceptable and very very nice implant. The electrode is passed through the saphenous or the femoral vein and then is implanted in the right lower quadrant. Special electrodes were made by CPI and we'll be starting to employ some of these other types of techniques. I am sure you will see that in the literature in the future from Dr. Udall.

QUESTION

Hilbert J. Th. Thalen, M.D.: Do you use atrial pacing in patients with IHSS?

RESPONSE

John Messenger, M.D.: No, we have not done it on a permanent basis. We have done it on a temporary basis using sequential ventricular pacing and an echocardiographic technique in various portions of the ventricle. This study entails ventricular pacing and then atrial pacing using a temporary electrode placed in the coronary sinus or placed in the atrium. The study is performed in the cardiovascular laboratory and cardiac outputs and imaging in the left anterior oblique view are done. We record anterior mitral leaflet motion and septal wall motion, and we have studied two cases. The results are not conclusive, and we are really not prepared to permanently atrial pace these people at the present.

QUESTION

Victor Parsonnet, M.D.: Do you have long term thresholds with coronary sinus pacing?

RESPONSE

John Messenger, M.D.: I made the earlier comment that we had had the same experience which was published in 1970 by Dr. Moss. His rise in threshold was 1.0 m.a. Ours was 1.5 m.a. The average life of our pacemakers is a little bit under 23 months, although some are as old as 6 or 7 years. The average change in threshold was about 1.5 m.a. So we can say that it appears to be reasonable. We generally accept 3.0 m.a. or less for initial implant.

QUESTION

Richard Coskey, M.D. (St. Joseph's Medical Center, Burbank, California): Have you had experience with patients who have done poorly with ventricular stimulators but who have done better or have been improved with atrial pacing?

RESPONSE

J. Warren Harthorne, M.D.: My own personal answer is an emphatic yes. I showed one of them earlier of a lady who developed pacemaker induced hypotension. We have had three such patients documented in the catheter laboratory with intra arterial recordings who, during the onset of ventricular stimulation, developed profound hypotension which was avoided by changing over to atrial stimulation. My clinical experience as a cardiologist of following 40 or 50 survivors beyond eight years of ventricular stimulation is that a rather large number of them ultimately end up on digitalis and diuretics. I suspect this would not be a problem in many if they had either atrial stimulation or AV synchronous stimulation.

John Messenger, M.D.: Most of our experience is anecdotal. We have had a patient with a bipolar ventricular pacemaker, a patient who was in congestive heart failure. An atrial electrode was placed in the patient, and he improved dramatically. There was no other change in therapy, and a spontaneous diuresis occurred with the return of atrial kick. And I think we have done enough with temporary atrio-ventricular pacing to support the hypothesis that return of atrial transport helps the patient out for a significant period of time and improves their lifestyle. Whether or not it prolongs life is unknown.

Hilbert J. Th. Thalen, M.D.: I should like to add a word. Larsen of Sweden has said to us, 'I almost don't need followup, because when the atrial triggered pacemaker gets a decrease of the battery voltage, it reverts to a fixed rate mode, and patients are aware of that change.' I think that tells you that there is really a difference for some patients between an atrial triggered unit and a fixed rate one.

J. Warren Harthorne, M.D.: Dr. Parsonnet has a comment.

Victor Parsonnet, M.D.: Yes, I would like to make a comment about the technique of putting these electrodes in. The coronary sinus technique is one method of using the atrium, and we have heard a lot of that today. I agree with the importance of the atrium. It's particularly important, of course, following open heart surgery, but it's also very important in patients with impaired ventricular function who need every bit of the atrial kick. Dr. Zucker and I have used the atrial appendage with the American Optical J-shaped electrode and have put in 41 of them. The cumulative survival data on these electrodes indicates that at about 5 years, only 75 percent will still be functioning. Many of them are lost for reasons of late threshold rise and sensing problems. Our early dislodgements were only two, about 4-$\frac{1}{2}$ percent; so, it's an acceptable technique if done properly. I think we should for completeness and thoroughness at this meeting remember that there are other ways of performing atrial pacing. One includes the method of Dr. Udall which he has published before, but I didn't know that he had ever used it in a patient until now. Carlton, I think, made a small incision to the right of the sternum and placed the electrode directly onto the atrium. The use of the esophagus is another possibility, and of course the technique that is used very frequently in Europe is the insertion of an electrode through a medias-tinoscope against the atrium. I am certain that Dr. Thalen and perhaps others on the panel can report on that use, but it might be appropriate to hear about it before leaving this topic.

Hilbert J. Th. Thalen, M.D.: We have implanted eight to ten units so far by mediastinoscopy. The mediastinoscopy electrode, made by Siemens Elema, is an ideal electrode for sensing, but is a very difficult electrode for stimulating. You can have a nice atrial triggered unit, but it is very difficult for bifocal demand pacing or for stimulation of the atrium. So far we have had one difficulty where the electrode slipped a little bit back. Larsen in Goteborg, Sweden has a large experience of over 200 cases with a long followup of about 6-8 years. He has warned that one of the troubles you might observe in some instances is that the electrode which has been placed by mediastinoscopy may slip back with re-sultant rise in threshold. In our experience with this method, the P-waves show an amplitude between 2 and 4 millivolts.

QUESTION
Igor Palacios, M.D. (Caracas, Venezuela): Could you elaborate on how it may be possible for the pacemaker circuit to regulate its own rate of stimulation by a biologic feedback mechanism?

RESPONSE
David L. Bowers, B.S.E.E.: In my earlier remarks I tried to make a parallelism between the externally programmable system and what could be achieved in the future by making it more automatic or self regulated. I tthink the limitation of such a system is really the type of sensor that is necessary to pick up this infor-mation. As yet, we have not been able to use a physiologic response mechanism in the heart to regulate the rate. Dr. Irnich pointed out that attempts have been made to use respiration to provide some regulatory means for rate. I don't know what the solution will be. Through proper investigation and proper insight into sensing mechanisms and also by working very closely with the physiologists and using information derived in the future from advanced monitoring technique, we may be able to find a solution. There are a number of techniques which can be employed, and at the present time we are using electrical phenomena determin-ing the evoked response as Dr. Preston indicated. There are also pressor in-dicators and other sensors that will be considered in the future.

Josef K. Cywinski, Ph.D.: I want to add to the scope Dave presented. At the recent pacemaker congress in Tokyo, there was a paper on this very subject delivered by Dr. Camilli from Florence, Italy. He has built a pacemaker with a controllable rate in which the controlling factor was pH. PH electrodes were placed on the endocardial catheter lead itself. He reports that he has six months' experience on human implants, and he is very pleased with this development of physiological rate control with pH electrodes in the bloodstream.

QUESTION

Joseph Amato, M.D. (New England Medical Center, Boston, Mass.): What about pacemakers for children; are there any new trends in size, programmability, high rate, and what is the current thought about the radio frequency pacemaker?

RESPONSE

J. Warren Harthorne, M.D.: I don't think any of us has had very much experience with this. It is curious that the solution has not arisen. Radiofrequency pacing was introduced by William Glenn years ago. The reports in the literature from Walter Gamble and from the group in Gainesville are noted primarily for the remarkable frequency of complication. These children are falling out of trees, off bicycles, and whatnot, breaking their electrodes, becoming septic, and have horrendous complications. My own personal experience includes one patient in fifteen years, an infant flown in from Maine with a functioning temporary wire with congenital heart block who died when the temporary pacemaker fell off the side of the bed and the electrode dislodged. I don't have other personal experience but I would like to make that an open question to the people on the panel.

Hilbert J. Th. Thalen, M.D.: We have one patient that was operated for a primum ASD and had to be paced later on. She is now going for about three years, and we had a lot of complications. Mostly in these children the complications are with the electrodes. Most electrodes have been designed for large hearts. In the smaller children's hearts, intramural or corkscrew electrodes can cause some trouble. The hearts move faster, but what's also very important is that the heart is small so, relative to the electrode, the movements are larger. A french group implants the pacemaker in the abdominal area with epicardial electrodes and they claim that they have not too much trouble. Our own experience with children is small but it seems that implants in the abdominal area for this group give better results than implants in the thoracic area. There is also the problem of the growth of the children as they get older which puts tension on the electrode wire.

J. Warren Harthorne, M.D.: Another approach which I have read is from a group in California in which AV synchronous wires and the generator are implanted in the thoracic cavity. Apparently this becomes rapidly walled off so that at a subsequent generator change, one can remove the rib overlying the generator. It sounds horrendous, but the experience was in about 14 children and was reported some years ago. It was a rather remarkable series. Dr. Parsonnet, do you have any experiences in infant pacing?

Victor Parsonnet, M.D.: No, really none. We have one youngster now, but our practice is mostly geriatrics. A paper that Dr. Furman wrote on about 38 children with pacemakers indicated that the complications are very frequent, particularly with electrode fractures. I would like to make a comment about the abdominal position of the pacemaker. We must differentiate between infant pacers in the new born and the first two or three years of life, and those in children who are ten and eleven. Abdominal implants appear superficially like a good idea, but they are not necessarily so because of the difficulty in taking out the generator sooner or later. It's a big operation to get it out when it's lying retropiretoneally above the kidney, and it doesn't take away any problems. It doesn't affect the wire fractures. You mentioned before that R-F pacers of Bill Glenn. This, of course, for an infant who is very active, is a bad idea. Dr. Camilli and many different others did it before. I would personally go to the smallest pacemaker I could find and do it transvenously and every now and then when the child grew enough, I would open the pocket and push a little more of that wire down into the heart.

QUESTION

Maximiliaan Kaulbach, M.D. (Salem Hospital, Salem, Mass.): What parameters should be measured and how, when implanting a permanent pacemaker system? How do you test for sensitivity in demand pacemaker devices?

RESPONSE

Paul Axelrod, M.D. (invited guest speaker, cardiologist, Beth Israel Hospital, Boston, Mass.): The measurement of impedance is really not a difficult measurement. Using Ohm's Law you have three parameters which are related, the voltage of the impulse, the current of the impulse and by Ohm's Law the third factor, that is the impedance or resistance of the patient's electrode system. So by Ohm's Law, if you know the current threshold, and if you divide that into the voltage threshold, you have impedance. The measurement of sensitivity with pacemakers is a terribly complicated subject. To do it effectively, you must have direct connections to the pacing device. The sensitivity of the system is partly related to the catheter connected to the device, and that has to be taken into account. The sensitivity is different depending upon the type of wave form that is used to measure the sensitivity, and there is very little agreement in the industry as to what kind of wave form should be used. You can imagine that when you are trying to simulate a normal QRS with a duration of .06 or .08 seconds and at the same time encompass the QRS which has a duration of .16 seconds, it becomes a little difficult to have agreement as to what is an ideal signal for testing sensitivity. The study of this is still in its infancy and that is part of the topic with which national standards are about. You don't eliminate sensing problems really by having a nicely designed pacemaker which is high in sensitivity. It is the combination of electrode and generator that has to be dealt with.

Hilbert, J. Th. Thalen, M.D.: I should like to make one comment on the measurement of the resistance. I think it can be dangerous to measure the resistance from the threshold data because the resistance in the electrode system is a complex one. It relates to the electrode but also the polarization surrounding the tip of the electrode and polarization can go as high as 1.5 volts. That means that when you have a 6 volts stimulus, about one quarter of the resistance can be due to polarization around that electrode tip. Another thing that can influence the resistance of your system is the choice of the second electrode. When it is a large one, it has low resistance; when it is a small one, it has a high resistance. So to measure exactly the resistance and to do it reproduceably, you have to measure the resistance at the same voltage that you did before, and if possible with the same indifferent electrode. When you do it with the same voltage, you have a big chance that you have the same polarization. However, when you measure the first time and find the stimulation threshold is 0.5 to 1.0 volts and the next time you find 0.3 volts, you probably have a change in the polarization voltage, and this will give you another resistance. You are anxious to know what changes in the resistance of the wire may have occurred in order that you may assess its integrity. You can only perform these measurements accurately when you have the same voltage and then you can read off the current or reverse.

Paul Axelrod, M.D.: I think you ha e to view this as really two separate problems. From a clinical standpoint, we are interested in whether the number of volts supplied by the output circuit of a particular generator is adequate to pace a particular patient. I am less interested in whether the impedance to electron flow is at the interface or whether it is within the electrode itself. The impedance which I have talked about is one I think which better summarizes the patient electrode system and which permits you to extrapolate in practical terms as to whether the generator really will or will not function on a particular patient. Not only does the impedance change as a function of polarization but it also changes as a function of time into the impulse and with the particular morphology of the impulse. It is truly a very complicated factor.

Hilbert J. Th. Thalen, M.D.: That's true. It's important to learn if the system is still intact or not. We have all seen systems that function properly but are defective. I agree, of course, that resistance is related to pulse width and to the type of stimulus you are giving. There has been a lot of research done into various impulse shapes. What's the best shape? It appears that the leading edge is very important and particularly its steepness. However, to get a very fast increase in the leading edge, you need a special electrode-circuit system that is almost impossible to make electronically without losing too much energy. I think we should be happy with what we have now.

QUESTION
Victor Parsonnet, M.D.: In a clinical setting, particularly in long life pacemakers, the type of heart block, and arrhythimas tend to change. Why isn't the ideal pacemaker an atrial and ventricular synchronized sequential pacemaker for everyone?

RESPONSE
Werner Irnich, M.D.: Yes, I would say that is the real ideal pacemaker. One type, instead of four different types, only one which is capable of restoring in the best way every disease of the heart, and this would be in my opinion the ideal pacemaker.

QUESTION
J. Warren Harthorne, M.D.: Dr. Zoll, with your background of twenty years of cardiac pacing techniques, do you perceive the recent introduction of such refinements as hermetic sealing, external programmability, hybrid circuitry, etc., as important developments or just frosting on the cake? Is the industry outstripping the needs and the requirements of the average patient?

RESPONSE
Paul M. Zoll, M.D.: My experience has been such a long and sad one, that I am still fixed on the need for reliability which still has not reached what I consider a satisfactory level. The reliability of the pacemaker system involves both the electrode and the pulse generator, and I am for any change that will improve reliability. I hope I am not so old and fossilized that I don't like change. I do agree that the integrated circuitry that is now becoming available permits us to use multiple components without multiplying the unreliability of each individual component as used to be the case. It is still not clear to me, however, that we have reached that stage in clinical application. I agree that hermetic sealing is a very important concept to improve the reliability of the power source. I think that one can probably use hermetic sealing even with mercury zinc batteries if one pro-

vides space inside of the can evacuated to a vacuum so that there is room for gas formation without causing trouble. I don't think one needs a lithium cell to permit hermetic sealing. I think you can do hermetic sealing even with a battery source that involves gas production. I am still not ready to use lithium cells because I haven't seen long enough in vivo experience with them. I think that the major cause for my reluctance to embrace the new changes with enthusiasm is the long observation we have had of how many new things that have been introduced over the last umteen years that looked very fine for the first year and the second year and then failed. The major lesson is that it takes two or three years for built in changes to produce built in new failure modes. That's why I think we should not go on to accept new procedures until they have had a chance either in the laboratory or in the hands of other bolder clinical investigators with their patients, not with mine, to prove that they are indeed safe. Once this has been done, I will accept rather belatedly new power sources, more useful programmable systems and so on. I think the tracking system that was suggested offers exciting possibilities that permit us to know where the threshold is and where the voltage output is and so on without intervention, and that's great, but somebody has to prove to me that it's safe and will work without additional problems for a matter of two or three years. This goes back to the repeated experiences we saw years ago when some people were presenting every year changes in their systems which had obvious advantages if we could only believe they were reliable. Every year they would come out with one year's experience with this system or another and so much better than what they had before. Well the one year's improvement is not satisfactory. You have to wait two or three years or more.

Paul Axelrod, M.D.: Dr. Zoll, how many units do you have to watch for how many years before you are reasonably satisfied with a system that it is reliably worthy?

Paul M. Zoll, M.D.: Well, I think you have to watch somewhere between 25 and 50 units for at least two or three years.

David L. Bowers. B.S.E.E.: I would like to make a comment on how the pacemaker business has matured in the past fifteen years. We are reaching levels of sophistication, and we cannot afford to make mistakes. I do want to offer an observation or suggestion of how we may overcome this period of time between a new idea or an improvement being implemented and actually being accepted. I don't think we can wait for final results, especially if you are talking of power sources that are going to last for ten years. We can't wait ten years to decide whether this is going to be accepted or not. But ther are some interesting possibilities in the field of acceleration testing of pacemaker devices to provide a good performance profile of what to anticipate. That doesn't mean that we'll completely replace testing in vivo, but it will give us a good insight into failure modes. Through this method of accelerated stressing of the pacemaker system in vitro to achieve the best performance and then moving on to the in vivo testing, we can come to some answers very quickly without being subjected to many surprises.

QUESTION

J. Warren Harthorne, M.D.: There is a question here which is a very practical one and comes from Dr. Howard Corning of Falmouth, Cape Cod and pertains to the measurement of stimulation threshold at the time of the procedure. We have been hearing from people who are talking about doing 1,000 pacemaker implants. We have done something like 3 or 4,000 generator changes at the Massachusetts General Hospital. Dr. Parsonnet's experience has probably doubled that. You have heard from engineers who have written textbooks, are knowledgeable in the electronics field and have thrown these figures around as if there is nothing to it. But what about the community hospital that may be doing 25 to 30 implants per year or 50 pacemaker implants per year? Oscilloscopes, sophisticated testing devices and the measurement of lead impedance, may be ethereal and unavailable. What does one do when you only have a temporary pacemaker device that stimulates at a 2 millisecond pulse width? Can you measure a reliable stimulation threshold at the time of the generator change? The question is directed to me. I am not smart enough to answer it. So I am going to ask Dr. Thalen.

RESPONSE

Hilbert J. Th. Thalen, M.D.: I am not smart enough to answer it either but I think when you only have an external unit, you shouldn't start implanting permanent pacers. You really need to have an external unit that enables you, at various impulse durations, to measure the current and the voltage thresholds. The other question you have from Dr. Corning of Falmouth is: Can we, from the power threshold, predict adequacy of the pulse generator with a variable pulse width? We cannot because power threshold is the current multiplied by the voltage multiplied by the time, and for these measurements to predict something we will have to make the measurement at the output pulse width of the pacemaker. So, I would say to everybody, make careful measurements of voltage and current when you start to implant pacemakers, and at the pulse width of the unit you are going to use.

J. Warren Harthorne, M.D.: The answer to Dr. Corning is that he has to get one of his well-to-do patients to buy him a variable pulse width stimulator.

QUESTION

J. Warren Harthorne, M.D.: The last question which I would like to address to the entire panel is the following: In 1975 it was estimated that in the world 150,000 pacemaker devices were employed. This was for both primary insertion and for generator replacement. That may be erroneous by a few thousand, but take for example, 150,000 pulse generators per year. We have now a family of energy sources which range from the mercury zinc RM1 Group 2 cell, the new lithium saft, the 702E Greatbatch cells, the ARCO lithiums, the rechargeable Pacesetter nickel cadmium units, the Biotronik beta cell stimulators and the plutonium powered nuclear devices and Dr. Cywinski's Biogalvanic. If we look at the commercial price range of those pacemaker devices, the mercury zinc powered fixed rate pacemaker is approximately $ 900 and going up. The demand mercury zinc pacemaker is approximately $ 1200 – $ 1500, depending upon whether it is programmable. The lithiums begin at $ 1800 and go on to $ 2200. The beta cell is $ 3300 and a little higher I guess now. I think the rechargeable Pacesetter is about $ 2600 and the plutoniums are now going up toward $ 6,000. Consider for the moment the mercury zinc demand pacemaker at $ 1200 and a lithium pacemaker at $ 2200. The difference for the world economy annually of 150,000 pacemakers is approximately $ 150,000,000. I would ask the panelists if they would respond to the following question. Does the mercury zinc pacemaker have a future or will it be phased out entirely by lithium? Can we foresee from our clinical projections of 27% of our patients being dead in two years and 50% of them being dead in five years that there will always be a role for mercury zinc pacemakers.

RESPONSE

Thomas Preston, M.D.: That's something like predicting the stock market I think. My opinion is that the longer lived units are economically justified because these units go five to six years and prevent re-operations. I think that there will always be a place for the mercury zinc at least for the next five or ten years; for the low cost unit for instance for the underdeveloped countries, or situations where the initial cost is really important. The usual case for this country is for the cost to be covered by third party carriers.

Victor Parsonnet, M.D.: I would answer the question by saying that the objective I would have for a patient is to give him a lifetime pacemaker because I don't know what that lifetime will be even in a patient with congestive failure who is 80. I therefore wish to give him a pacemaker that will last as long as possible. With all the problems of the mercury zinc over the years, despite its improvements in view of the fact that it is difficult to hermetically seal and in view of the recent experience with lithium units with no battery failures in almost four years, I would think that the mercury zinc cell is going to be gone a lot sooner than five or ten years.

David L. Bowers, Ph.D.: I would like to comment just from a technical stand-point. The mercury zinc cell now has a number of improvements that have been implemented and a number that have been suggested. The question is will the suggested improvements of the mercury zinc cell be implemented if there isn't motivation on the part of the battery manufacturer. I think that the mercury zinc system will have a place; where it is in terms of numbers will have to come from the medical profession. Technically, it can be very nicely worked into a family of products.

Werner Irnich, Ph.D.: The cost of pacemaker implantation is not only given by the pacemaker cost but also by the implantation costs, and this is the reason why life long pacemakers in any case are the cheapest. If you have to implant two pacemakers, it's in every case the most expensive and therefore the problem is to look for a pacemaker which just lasts one month longer than the patient. This solution of this problem would be the best one. Now I am convinced that with conventional mercury oxide batteries we will reach five or six years; with lithium batteries we may obtain more than ten years. The 50% survival time lies between five and seven years, depending on sex. I would say if 60% of all patients would have a lithium pacemaker, and 40% of the conventional one, then perhaps this would be a system of the lowest costs.

Paul M. Zoll, M.D.: Our experience with the pacemakers we have been using lately with a relatively low drain, particularly with a short stimulus duration, suggests to us that the mercury zinc pacemakers can and are lasting well over three years, into their fourth year and some nearly five years. I think we will continue to use these same pacemakers even though they are a little complicated because we have had such a good experience with them until we see that the lithium pacemaker does indeed do better for longer periods of time. I think if we can have a mercury zinc system that lasts four years or so, there will always be a place for such a pulse generator.

Josef K. Cywinski, Ph.D.: I will have to agree with all of the previous speakers. I must say that experience is the best school there is as Henry Ford said, except its graduates are sometimes too old to work, and that is what is happening to mercury zinc cells. The lithium cell is coming on the horizon. It is not yet ap-parent that it will phase out mercury; it will have to prove itself. However, the probability of success with lithium is much higher than mercury zinc cells be-cause of different failure modes and different internal construction and the inherent high reliability ability of lithium cells, we may have some other cells on the market which may provide a true lifetime pacemaker for every patient.

Paul Axelrod, M.D.: I have a feeling that we are not going to stop at lithium either. Somehow the problems always resolve themselves and science moves forward. There is a tremendous craze in this world of ours at the present time to be concerned about pacemaker survival, and I continually claim that the emphasis must always be on patient survival. If you could manufacture for me a pacemaker that would work exactly six years reliably where you did not have to worry about the energy source at any time during that six years, that to me would be a very desirable pacemaker regardless of the power source. If you offered a pacemaker to me that would run somewhere between seven and ten years, I would say that is not as desirable. I am much more concerned about the safety of my patients than I am the number of times he is operated on, and I think that the reliability with which it produces that long life is more important than duration of function. Unfortunately, there is no rapid technique of assessing the manner in which a device will survive three years and then to predict the way in which it will deteriorate at end of life. The only real test is the test of time. That is, in the case of lithium, we are going to have to wait somewhere between another three and ten or fifteen years to see just what is going to happen at the outside end of these devices. Lithium is very exciting because it certainly suggests an advance in both reliability and certainly in longevity, but if we find out that lithium is less predictable in the last half of its life, then I will not be dissatisfied with mercury zinc and will continue using it. In following about 300 patients in the usual fashion which we do, where we have virtually all mercury zinc pacemakers, we have not had one death in three years which I can attribute to unpredictable battery operation. It's not ideal and pacemakers do not function for an ideal length of time, but certainly in terms of patient survival, I think it has been very safe.

John Messenger, M.D.: Our experience with mercury zinc has been very satisfactory. With the special interest pacers we have gone into we have been more concerned about performance and reliability than we have about long term function and therefore we've looked for those factors somewhat like Dr. Zoll mentioned, but I would be in agreement with what Paul Axelrod has to say in terms of his experience. Probably we'll see a mix of lithium and mercury for a while with the winner being determined by the end stage reliability of lithium.

Hilbert J. Th. Thalen, M.D.: So much as been said, and I can only add a little bit. I think by now that there are about 150,000 pacemakers implanted a year worldwide. It is very difficult to predict what will be the lifetime of the pacemaker patient, and we have all tried to give the patient a lifetime pacemaker. The least expensive device would be one which would cease to function one week after the patient's death. That is almost impossible. We have heard that diabetes is a high risk. One of our patients had his pacemaker implanted on the 21st of March 1963 and was a diabetic. He is still doing fine. It is very difficult. You can make rough outlines. Another thing which is very important and which we have to think about is that the epoxy resin allows penetration of fluid. When you leave a pacemaker in a patient, it always happier when you take it out. When pacemakers last longer, you may be sure that sooner or later fluid will reach the circuit. Therefore, when you speak about long lasting pacemakers, you have to talk about hermetically sealed pacemakers. It is a pity, but mercury zinc cells cannot be hermetically sealed because they produce gas. One of the features of lithium is that not only that it has a nice life expectancy, but they also enable us to make a hermetically sealed circuitry and energy source. By now there are five different lithium batteries on the market, five various chemical energy sources, all working with lithium. I agree that in the future you will see other energy sources. In Tokyo, Greatbatch made a guess, and I think that could be a real nice guess, that there will always be mercury zinc cells. Lithium may, in about three years; account for 40% of the market, perhaps a little bit more, and then there may be a small place for the nuclear. So far there have been only 2500 nuclear pacemakers implanted worldwide. The availability of lithium has decreased that number and it is especially the paper work that is involved with the nuclear pacemakers; also the great size of these units may be a little bit troublesome. So in summary, lithium yes. We are shifting a little bit from the mercury zinc very carefully, because I think, Dr. Zoll, that at least some people should start with newer things.

J. Warren Harthorne, M.D.: Thank you. The question is really an economic as well as philosophical one that an economist should respond to because it pertains to the cost to the world economy of cardiac pacing. We are privileged to sit in a rather expensive hotel in a rather expensive city where third party carriers cover the medical cost of all of our patients. The economics of medical therapy seldom enters into performance of the procedures, but there are vast areas in the world in Southeast Asia, in India, and Africa where large numbers of patients are not receiving pacemakers simply because of the cost. It has been proposed that a low cost pacemaker device be made available for certain categories of patients. The answers are economic and philosophic and perhaps even to a certain extent religious. I promised to start the program on time and end on time, and my watch indicates that I have missed that by a few minutes. We've had a good day together, and we've enjoyed your comments and questions, and we thank you all for coming.

INDEX